Digital Medicine Starter Guide

Alfredo Cesario • Marco Gorini
Domenico D'Amario

Digital Medicine Starter Guide

Springer

Alfredo Cesario
Fondazione Policlinico Universitario
Agostino Gemelli IRCCS, GDMH -
Gemelli Digital Medicine & Health Srl
Rome, Italy

Marco Gorini
Innovation Unit & Business Excellence
Astrazeneca
Milano, Italy

Domenico D'Amario
Department of Traslational
Medicine (DIMET)
Università del Piemonte Orientale
Novara, Italy

ISBN 978-3-032-01271-5 ISBN 978-3-032-01272-2 (eBook)
https://doi.org/10.1007/978-3-032-01272-2

This Springer imprint is published by the registered company Springer Nature Switzerland AG
The registered company address is: Gewerbestrasse 11, 6330 Cham, Switzerland

To the pioneers—visionary professionals from diverse fields such as medicine, technology, data science, law, and beyond—who have courageously ventured beyond the traditional confines of their disciplines to shape the future of healthcare: your unwavering pursuit of innovation, your audacity to challenge established conventions, and your steadfast commitment to collaboration have culminated in the advent of Digital Medicine. This is not merely an extension of existing fields; rather, it is a self-standing endeavor and a transformative force that is reshaping Models of Care and, ultimately, serving as a bridge to improved health outcomes.

Above all, this work is dedicated to the patients—those who inspire every breakthrough, innovation, and effort to push the limits of what is possible. May Digital Medicine continue to serve as a powerful tool to enhance their lives, offering not merely treatment but understanding, empowerment, and hope.

Foreword

"Artificial intelligence should not be considered as a substitute for humans, since the sensitivity of the doctor and healthcare worker cannot be replaced"

In my professional journey—first as a physician and academic in the field of Nuclear Medicine and Molecular Imaging, and now as Minister of Health—I have witnessed the profound transformation of medicine through the responsible application of science and technology. These changes have not only advanced diagnostics and treatment but reshaped the very architecture of healthcare systems.

Digital Medicine stands today as one of the most strategic frontiers of innovation. It promises greater precision in diagnosis, earlier intervention, enhanced patient monitoring, and more personalized care. Furthermore, it introduces a new model of healthcare—more continuous, more proactive, and more focused on people's real needs. This evolution requires not only technological infrastructure but also cultural readiness, regulatory clarity, and multidisciplinary competence.

In this regard, the *Digital Medicine Starter Guide* represents a timely and valuable resource. It is not merely a technical manual, but a structured tool for clinicians, researchers, administrators, and policymakers alike. It helps translate innovation into daily practice, aligning technology with the clinical, ethical, and organizational demands of a modern health system.

From my experience in Nuclear Medicine, I know how vital it is to interpret complex signals—to see beyond what is visible, to anticipate what is not yet manifest. Digital Medicine, in many ways, offers us similar capabilities. It equips us to act earlier, to be more precise, to intervene with more impact—without ever forgetting that *behind every dataset is a human story.*

This is precisely why we must never reduce the transformation underway to a matter of algorithms or automation. As I have said publicly, artificial intelligence and digital tools must support, not replace, the irreplaceable clinical sensibility and judgment of healthcare professionals. The human presence remains the cornerstone of care.

This book contributes to that vision. It reminds us that innovation in health is not an end in itself but a means to serve people, protect their dignity, and enhance their lives. I welcome this work and encourage all readers—whether you are just starting or already deep into digital transformation—to use it as a guide, a reference, and a catalyst for action.

Minister of Health, the Italian Republic
Professor of Nuclear Medicine
and Former Rector
University of Rome "Tor Vergata"
Rome, Italy

Orazio Schillaci

Foreword

In my dual role as a physician and a legislator, I appreciate the powerful convergence between science, care, and policy. Medicine, at its best, is not simply the application of clinical knowledge—it is an act of service, stewardship, and vision. As we stand at the frontier of a new era, Digital Medicine challenges us to reimagine not only how we treat disease but also how we design preventive, participatory, and profoundly human health systems.

My clinical journey began in the operating theatre, in the immediacy of decisions that can save or change a life. Surgery taught me the irreplaceable value of precision, evidence, and trust. But it also revealed the limits of an episodic model of care—one that too often engages the patient only in moments of crisis. Through digital medicine, I have seen a complementary model that extends our capacity to monitor, anticipate, and intervene before illness manifests in irreversible ways. It is a model that empowers doctors and nurses, patients, caregivers, and entire communities.

As a Member of Parliament and author of legislative initiatives focused on Digital Therapeutics (Dtx), I have championed that healthcare innovation must be institutionalized, not left to chance or the market alone. Across Europe, we have seen promising steps: Germany's DiGA model, France's evolving reimbursement pathways, and Belgium's pilot programs. Italy cannot afford to trail behind. We must ensure that high-quality digital interventions—grounded in scientific evidence and regulated as medical devices—are recognized, reimbursed, and responsibly implemented within our national health system.

Digital Medicine is not about replacing the clinician. It is about augmenting human intelligence with machine learning, expanding diagnostic reach through AI, ensuring continuity of care through remote monitoring, and personalizing treatment through data. It is about shifting from generalized guidelines to precision care plans, from fragmented records to interoperable systems, from reactive models to predictive ecosystems. Above all, it is about enabling people to live longer, healthier, and more autonomous lives.

Yet this transformation is not automatic. It requires deliberate, coordinated action. We must define rigorous pathways for the validation of Dtx, build institutional competence within regulatory agencies, educate healthcare professionals to work confidently with digital tools, protect data with strong privacy frameworks that do not stifle innovation, and remain vigilant against digital divides that risk excluding those most in need.

This is why the *Digital Medicine Starter Guide* is so timely and necessary. It is not a theoretical treatise—it is a practical compass. It helps the clinician navigate the complexities of software as a medical device. It provides policymakers with a structured overview of the regulatory landscape. It supports the innovator in aligning technology with clinical need. It engages the administrator in fostering cultural change within institutions. It invites us all to ask what digital medicine can do and how we can do it well.

One of the qualities I most appreciate in this guide is its openness. It acknowledges that digital transformation is not linear. It respects the diversity of healthcare systems, the pace of regulatory change, and the cultural factors that shape patient engagement. It does not offer dogma, but direction. It presents case studies, exercises, and blueprints that readers can adapt to their context, turning knowledge into action.

The pandemic taught us that health systems must be agile, connected, and resilient. However, we cannot build such systems by returning to old paradigms. We must embrace the tools of our time with wisdom, courage, and humility. That is the promise of digital medicine—and it is also its challenge.

To those who will read this book—whether you are a clinician, a policymaker, a technologist, or a student—I say this: the future of healthcare is already in your hands. With each decision you make, you shape outcomes and culture. This guide will accompany you on that journey. Let it be a resource, a stimulus, and a reminder that innovation, when rooted in values, can truly serve the common good.

Let us build together a digital medicine that does not lose sight of the human person, integrates technology without sacrificing empathy, and transforms care not as an end in itself but as a renewed expression of our duty to protect, heal, and include.

Simona Loizzo

Member of the Parliament, the Italian Republic, President, Parliamentary Intergroup on Digital Health and Digital Therapies
Director, Department of Surgery
Annunziata Hospital
Cosenza, Italy

Preface

Digital Medicine at the Crossroads of Innovation and Equity

Healthcare is entering an era of profound transformation. At the intersection of cutting-edge technology and timeless principles of care, Digital Medicine represents a paradigm shift that redefines how health is understood, managed, and delivered. However, this shift is not without its challenges. As healthcare systems grapple with rising costs, increasing inequities, and evolving patient needs, Digital Medicine presents both a solution and a challenge: *Can innovation be deployed in ways that genuinely benefit everyone?*

This book examines that question. It aims to unravel the complexities of Digital Medicine, providing a holistic perspective that bridges the theoretical, practical, and ethical dimensions of this rapidly evolving field. Through a combination of evidence-based insights, real-world examples, and actionable strategies, it equips readers with the tools to navigate the opportunities and challenges of Digital Medicine.

Framing the Narrative

The structure of this book is deliberate, mirroring the journey of Digital Medicine itself—from foundational principles to practical tools, systemic challenges, and future possibilities.

Chapter 1 introduces the foundational principles of Digital Medicine, emphasizing the shift from reactive to proactive care. Predictive analytics, participatory care, and continuous engagement are not merely buzzwords—they constitute the philosophical backbone of this transformation. This chapter establishes a framework for understanding how Digital Medicine aligns with broader goals of equity, accessibility, and patient empowerment.

Building on these principles, Chaps. 2 and 3 explore the tools that bring Digital Medicine to life. These chapters highlight the technologies reshaping the healthcare landscape, from telemedicine platforms that expand access for underserved communities to AI algorithms that improve diagnostic accuracy. However, they also emphasize the necessity for clinical validation, interoperability, and patient trust—key themes that recur throughout the book.

Chapters 4 and 5 concentrate on the practical realities of adoption. These chapters explore the challenges of integrating digital tools into complex healthcare ecosystems, including cultural resistance, financial constraints, and data privacy issues. Through a combination of case studies and strategic frameworks, they provide a roadmap for overcoming these obstacles, ensuring that innovation leads to meaningful impact.

Chapter 6 introduces a sociological perspective to the broader analysis within the publication, emphasizing the significance of critically evaluating the social risks and equity concerns associated with Digital Medicine. By examining how evolving definitions of "value" shape healthcare systems, this chapter underscores the importance of foreseeing potential exclusions, algorithmic biases, and systemic disparities. It encourages reflection on how digital innovation can be harmonized not solely with economic efficiency but also with social sustainability, inclusiveness, and patient-centered care.

Finally, Chap. 7 provides an examination of prospective developments by thoroughly investigating emerging technologies such as bioelectronic medicine, big data analytics, and immersive platforms. These innovations offer a preview of future possibilities while concurrently raising essential questions regarding ethics, equity, and sustainability.

Rome, Italy — Alfredo Cesario
Innovation Unit & Business Excellence — Marco Gorini
Astrazeneca, Milano, Italy
Università del Piemonte Orientale — Domenico D'Amario
Novara, Italy

Acknowledgments

We extend our sincere thanks to Francesca Romana Lacroce, BSc, MBA, for her insightful authorship of Chap. 6. Her sociological perspective and economic expertise contributed essential depth to the discussion on equity and value in Digital Medicine.

We are also deeply grateful to the Springer editorial team, including Grant Weston and Mahalakshmi Sethish Babu, for their unwavering support and professionalism (and patience) throughout the editorial process, which proved invaluable for the realization of this volume.

Roma, Milano, Novara (Italy), June 25, 2025

Competing Interests The authors have no competing interests to declare that are relevant to the content of this manuscript. The views expressed in this book by Marco Gorini are those of the author and do not represent the views of AstraZeneca.

Contents

About the Authors

Alfredo Cesario is a distinguished physician, clinical researcher, and fervent advocate for the incorporation of technology into healthcare. With over 30 years of experience in clinical medicine and research, he has dedicated his career to enhancing patient outcomes through innovative methodologies and evidence-based practices.

As a distinguished authority in the rapidly advancing field of Digital Medicine, he has authored a significant number of articles and provided mentorship to healthcare professionals regarding the implementation of innovative tools, including telemedicine, remote patient monitoring, digitally enabled clinical decision support systems, wearable devices, and artificial intelligence.

His vast knowledge integrates conventional medical practices with the transforming digital environment, thereby delivering practical insights aimed at improving patient care and enhancing operational efficiency.

As Chief Executive Officer, he oversees Gemelli Digital Medicine & Health, a Digital Medicine enterprise (www.gdmh.it), established as a part of the initiatives of one of Europe's largest healthcare institutions and foremost research centers, the Policlinico Gemelli (www.policlinicogemelli.it), located in Rome, Italy, where he also serves as Digital Health Manager.

He is dedicated to knowledge dissemination and capacity building alongside his professional commitments. Influenced by both personal and professional experiences, he developed the Digital Medicine Starter Guide 1.0 as a practical resource intended to empower healthcare practitioners in confidently navigating and embracing digital tools.

When not engaged in professional responsibilities, he enjoys exploring the intersections of science, technology, and human health, as well as mentoring emerging leaders in the realms of medicine and research.

He is the author of more than 365 peer-reviewed scientific articles, primarily in the fields of surgical oncology, lung cancer, systems medicine, and digital medicine. Furthermore, he has edited multiple books concerning innovation, personalized medicine and artificial intelligence, systems biology and medicine, clinical practice, and digital transformation within healthcare.

He holds a license as a Visual Flight Rules (VFR) ultralight (UL) pilot and frequently traverses the skies.

Marco Gorini is an experienced professional at AstraZeneca (www.astrazeneca.com). In his role as Head of the Digital Health and Innovation in Italy, he has led numerous initiatives at the intersection of pharmaceutical research, patient engagement and digital innovation. With over a decade of experience in clinical development and healthcare strategy, he has established himself as a prominent advocate for the application of technology to improve patient outcomes and streamline pharmaceutical processes.

Throughout his career, Marco has served as a pivotal figure in bridging the divide between emerging digital solutions and tangible clinical applications. He nurtures collaboration with healthcare organizations, start-ups, and policymakers to guarantee that innovative concepts transform into impactful treatments. Deeply committed to patient-centered care, he has advocated for the implementation of predictive analytics, telehealth, and data-driven decision-making within pharmaceutical initiatives, facilitating the advancement of more personalized and efficient therapies.

Marco commits his time to mentoring aspiring healthcare professionals during his engagement with digital transformation and clinical collaboration. He is of the opinion that the future of medicine is contingent upon cross-functional expertise and open dialogue. As a co-author of the *Digital Medicine Starter Guide V1.0*, he amalgamates his substantial background in pharmaceutical research with a vision for a more integrated, technology-driven healthcare system that prioritizes patients.

Domenico D'Amario serves as an Associate Professor of Cardiovascular Medicine at the Università del Piemonte Orientale and is the Director of the Cardiac Intensive Care Unit at Ospedale Maggiore della Carità in Novara, Italy. His areas of expertise include advanced heart failure management, interventional cardiology, and translational cardiovascular research.

With a robust background in clinical and academic medicine, he has significantly contributed to the understanding of coronary artery disease, heart failure, and pioneering cardiovascular treatments. His research interests encompass the advancement of innovative medical devices and digital tools aimed at enhancing cardiovascular care. He has held the position of principal investigator in European-funded research projects that concentrate on digital health, interoperability, and the practical applications of real-world data in the field of cardiology.

He holds the position of Associate Local Editor for the *European Heart Journal* and serves as the Deputy Editor for *European Heart Journal—Case Reports* and other leading academic journals actively influencing discussions on advancements in cardiovascular health. He is a Fellow of the European Society of Cardiology (FESC) and is recognized as a leading figure in digital health initiatives, contributing to international committees dedicated to digital medicine and the implementation of artificial intelligence in the management of heart failure.

In addition to his academic and clinical responsibilities, he is committed to fostering interdisciplinary collaborations that connect medicine, technology, and patient care. His involvement in the *Digital Medicine Starter Guide v1.0 serves* as a testament to his dedication to providing healthcare professionals with the knowledge and tools necessary to adopt digital transformation in the realm of cardiovascular medicine.

Setting the Stage: Understanding Digital Medicine 1

Introduction

Digital Medicine is redefining healthcare by transforming how we diagnose, treat, and manage health conditions. No longer an abstract concept or distant promise, it has become a fundamental component of modern medicine, shaping the future of patient care. At its core, Digital Medicine integrates innovative digital tools and technologies into clinical practice, allowing healthcare professionals to provide more precise, efficient, and personalized care. From telemedicine consultations to wearable devices that monitor real-time physiological data, these innovations are not merely tools but catalysts for a healthcare revolution.

But with the rapid evolution of Digital Health solutions, a key question emerges: What exactly does "Digital Medicine" encompass—and just as importantly, what does it not? The distinction between clinically validated digital tools and general consumer wellness technologies is critical for both healthcare professionals and patients.

The *Digital Medicine Starter Guide v1.0* is crafted as a pragmatic ***roadmap*** for healthcare professionals seeking to navigate the swiftly evolving domain of Digital Medicine. This publication provides clinicians, administrators, and policymakers with the essential knowledge necessary for the effective assessment, adoption, and integration of digital solutions. Furthermore, it empowers professionals to rigorously distinguish authentic innovations from transient technological trends, thereby ensuring that digital transformation is *centered on patient care, backed by evidence, and clinically beneficial.*

Yet, it is important to clarify that Digital Medicine does not replace clinical expertise or the human touch that defines high-quality care. Rather, it is a powerful complement—a *toolkit* that, when applied thoughtfully, enhances clinical decision-making, strengthens patient engagement, and streamlines healthcare delivery.

This guide is structured to help you:

A. Cesario et al., *Digital Medicine Starter Guide*,
https://doi.org/10.1007/978-3-032-01272-2_1

1. *Define Digital Medicine* by outlining its scope, opportunities, and limitations.
2. *Critically evaluate digital solutions* to determine their validity, safety, and practical application in real-world settings.
3. *Bridge the gap between theory and practice by* incorporating digital tools into clinical workflows with case studies, real-world examples, and strategic frameworks.

Digital Medicine is not a static destination but an evolving field—one that demands adaptability, continuous learning, and a willingness to embrace technological progress.

The *Digital Medicine Starter Guide* aims to assist you in navigating this paradigm shift, integrating digital tools as a vital, responsible, and effective component of your practice. The goal is straightforward to enhance patient outcomes while upholding the highest standards of medical ethics and care quality.

What Is Digital Medicine and What Is Not?

Digital Medicine represents a fundamental shift in healthcare delivery. It leverages advanced digital technologies to enhance patient outcomes, improve accessibility, and optimize clinical workflows. However, fully understanding its role requires differentiating it from adjacent fields such as Digital Health, health IT, and consumer wellness technologies.

What Digital Medicine Is

Digital Medicine consists of clinically validated digital tools that are designed to diagnose, treat, and manage health conditions. These tools extend beyond traditional medicine, incorporating technologies that generate real-time, actionable insights while ensuring integration into existing clinical workflows.

Key Characteristics of Digital Medicine

1. *Clinically Validated*. Digital tools undergo rigorous scientific evaluations, demonstrating their efficacy and safety in improving health outcomes.
2. *Integrated into Clinical Workflows*. Digital Medicine solutions complement medical practice, enhancing (rather than replacing) clinical decision-making.
3. *Patient-Centered and Personalized*. Digital tools facilitate individualized treatment plans, supporting precision medicine and tailored interventions.
4. *Dynamic and evolving*. As technology advances, it continuously incorporates innovations such as AI-driven diagnostics, real-time biosensors, and predictive analytics.

Examples of Digital Medicine Ecosystems

1. Continuous glucose monitors for diabetes management, providing real-time data for both patients and clinicians.
2. AI-assisted imaging tools, helping radiologists detect early stage diseases such as cancer with greater accuracy.
3. Digital Therapeutics (DTx), offering evidence-based interventions for conditions such as depression, insomnia, or chronic pain.
4. Wearable ECG devices, enabling remote monitoring of cardiac rhythms to prevent complications in high-risk patients.

What Digital Medicine Is Not

While Digital Medicine is a critical subset of Digital Health, it is distinct from consumer wellness apps, general health IT systems, and unregulated tools. Understanding these differences ensures that healthcare professionals *prioritize clinical-grade solutions* over products with unverified claims.

Digital Medicine Does Not Include

1. General Consumer Wellness Apps and Devices. Step counters, meditation apps, and basic fitness trackers do not qualify as Digital Medicine because they lack clinical validation and medical-grade accuracy.
2. Standalone Telemedicine Without Decision Support. While telemedicine facilitates virtual consultations, it only qualifies as Digital Medicine when integrated with clinical support tools (e.g., AI-powered diagnostics and remote monitoring).
3. Health IT systems (EHRs, scheduling tools, etc.) serve as the foundation for Digital Medicine, which concentrates on generating actionable insights rather than simply storing or organizing data.
4. Unregulated, Non-Evidence-Based Digital Solutions. Any app or device without regulatory approval (FDA, MDR, etc.) or clinical validation cannot be considered Digital Medicine.

Digital Medicine vs. Digital Health

Understanding where Digital Medicine fits within the broader Digital Health ecosystem is essential.

Term Definitions

Digital Health. A broad term encompasses all digital technologies that enhance health, including public health tools, wellness apps, and health IT systems.

Digital Medicine. A subset of Digital Health that focuses on clinically validated tools used directly in patient care.

Why Digital Medicine Matters for Healthcare Professionals and the Public

Digital Medicine is not merely a technological upgrade; it is a fundamental transformation of healthcare that impacts how patients engage with their health, how clinicians make decisions, and how healthcare systems operate at scale.

At its core, Digital Medicine represents a shift from episodic, reactive care—where medical interventions occur after symptoms manifest—to a proactive, continuous, and patient-centered model, where diseases can be detected earlier, prevented more effectively, and managed with greater precision. This shift is made possible by real-time data analytics, remote monitoring, artificial intelligence (AI), and interoperability—concepts explored in Chaps. 3, 4, and 5.

While Chap. 3 provides an in-depth analysis of the technologies enabling Digital Medicine—including wearables, mHealth apps, and AI-driven decision support—and Chap. 4 delves into the operational and implementation strategies, this section examines this evolving field's broader clinical, societal, and regulatory implications.

Empowering Patients and the Public

Traditionally, patients have been passive healthcare recipients, reliant on clinical visits, physician evaluations, and retrospective symptom reporting. Digital Medicine fundamentally alters this dynamic, placing individuals at the center of their healthcare journeys by enabling real-time engagement with their health status, data-driven self-management, and personalized interventions.

This shift aligns with the P4 Medicine model (Predictive, Preventive, Personalized, and Participative), which was first introduced in Chap. 2. This model emphasizes personalized and proactive care strategies.

Key Benefits of Empowering Patients

Continuous Health Monitoring

Wearable devices, biosensors, and Digital Health platforms enable patients to monitor their heart rate variability, glucose levels, blood pressure, and other crucial health indicators in real time.

Example. Continuous Glucose Monitors (CGMs) enable individuals with diabetes to track fluctuations in glucose levels, reducing complications and empowering lifestyle-based interventions.

(See Chap. 3.3 on wearables and biosensors for more on real-time patient monitoring.)

AI-Driven Symptom Tracking and Decision Support

mHealth applications provide real-time feedback and early alerts based on machine learning algorithms that analyze patient-reported symptoms.

Example. AI-powered chatbots assist individuals in triaging their symptoms, recommending home management, pharmacist consultations, or urgent care referrals based on severity.

(Refer to Chap. 3.2 on mHealth applications and Chap. 6.5.2 on AI-driven patient education.)

Enhanced Health Literacy and Self-Management

AI-powered virtual assistants translate complex medical information into personalized, actionable insights, ensuring better patient comprehension and adherence to treatment plans.

Example. An app for hypertension management that visualizes blood pressure trends suggests lifestyle modifications and provides educational content based on patient behaviors.

(See Chap. 6.5.1 on informed decision-making.)

Equitable Access to Specialized Care

Telemedicine removes geographical, financial, and logistical barriers to care, allowing rural populations, older adults, and individuals with limited mobility to access specialist consultations.

Example. A rural cardiac patient can consult a specialist via telehealth while wearing a remote ECG patch that transmits real-time cardiovascular data.

(See Chap. 3.1 on telemedicine and Chap. 5.3 on digital equity.)

Despite these benefits, barriers to adoption persist, including digital literacy challenges, privacy concerns, and accessibility issues. These obstacles are addressed in Chap. 5, where strategies to enhance trust, bridge the digital divide, and promote digital literacy are discussed.

Elevating Clinical Practice

Digital Medicine introduces a paradigm shift for healthcare professionals in how patient data is collected, analyzed, and applied to clinical decision-making. Rather than relying solely on intermittent clinical assessments and patient-reported symptoms, providers now have access to continuous, real-time data streams that enable them to proactively manage conditions, anticipate complications, and intervene earlier.

Key Benefits for Clinicians

AI-Augmented Clinical Decision-Making

AI-powered clinical decision support systems (CDSS) analyze vast datasets to identify patterns, early warning signs, and optimal treatment strategies.

AI-assisted radiology tools detect microscopic tumor growth in imaging scans, offering early stage cancer detection and tailored oncology recommendations.

(See Chap. 3.4 on AI in clinical practice and Chap. 6.2 on big data analytics.)

Predictive and Preventive Care Strategies

Digital tools allow for risk stratification, predictive analytics, and personalized prevention plans.

Example. Cardiac patients equipped with wearable ECG monitors receive AI-generated alerts for arrhythmias or potential heart failure exacerbations, allowing preventive intervention.

(See Chap. 4.6 on measuring impact and Chap. 6.2.1 on predictive analytics for population health.)

Operational Efficiency and Streamlined Workflows

AI-driven tools automate routine tasks (e.g., documentation, triaging, scheduling), reducing administrative burdens.

Example. AI-powered voice transcription tools integrate with Electronic Health Records (EHRs) to document real-time clinical encounters.

(See Chap. 4.3 on EHR integration and Chap. 5.1.2 on overcoming clinician resistance.)

Despite these advantages, workforce adaptation, regulatory oversight, and reimbursement challenges remain significant barriers to adoption. These issues are examined in Chap. 5, where strategies to overcome implementation hurdles are outlined.

Innovation with Regulation

As Digital Medicine becomes deeply embedded in healthcare, regulatory frameworks must evolve to balance innovation, safety, and privacy.

Key Regulatory Considerations

As Digital Medicine becomes increasingly embedded in healthcare, regulatory frameworks must evolve to balance *innovation, safety, and privacy*. Unlike traditional pharmaceuticals or medical devices, digital tools often operate in real-time, continuously collecting, processing, and analyzing patient data. This dynamic nature introduces *new regulatory challenges*, from ensuring clinical validation to safeguarding sensitive health information.

One of the most pressing concerns is *clinical validation and safety*. To ensure that digital tools deliver meaningful health benefits without introducing risk, regulatory frameworks worldwide require rigorous evidence demonstrating efficacy and reliability. AI-driven diagnostics, for instance, must undergo extensive testing to ensure they provide accurate recommendations across diverse patient populations. Without such oversight, the integration of digital tools into medical workflows could lead to inconsistent outcomes, algorithmic biases, or unintended clinical consequences.

In addition to clinical efficacy, the importance of data privacy and cybersecurity cannot be overstated. Given the significant amounts of patient data circulating through digital platforms, the General Data Protection Regulation (GDPR) in Europe, the Health Insurance Portability and Accountability Act (HIPAA) in the United States, and similar regulations across the globe establish comprehensive guidelines for data collection, storage, and sharing. These frameworks ensure that patient information is managed in accordance with the highest security standards while affording individuals enhanced control over their personal health data. The introduction of the European Health Data Space (EHDS) represents a substantial advancement in this area, aiming to standardize cross-border data exchange while upholding stringent privacy protections. It is anticipated to take effect during the 2027–2028 biennium.

In addition to safety and privacy considerations, the economic sustainability of Digital Medicine is contingent upon the establishment of well-defined reimbursement models that promote adoption while substantiating real-world value. Numerous healthcare systems continue to function under antiquated payment structures that fail to accommodate remote patient monitoring, digital therapeutics, or AI-driven diagnostics. Consequently, hospitals and clinics frequently encounter financial obstacles when attempting to integrate digital tools into standard care. Nevertheless, value-based reimbursement models are emerging, whereby insurers and healthcare providers align payments with quantifiable enhancements in patient outcomes. For instance, hospitals that implement Remote Patient Monitoring (RPM) for heart failure patients can negotiate contracts predicated on the reduction of hospital readmissions, thereby demonstrating cost savings and improved clinical outcomes.

As Digital Medicine continues to evolve, global collaboration between regulators, policymakers, and industry leaders will be crucial. The challenge is to develop adaptive regulations that keep pace with innovation while maintaining patient safety and ethical integrity. In this rapidly shifting landscape, balancing technological progress with responsible oversight will determine the long-term success and trustworthiness of Digital Medicine.

Example: The European Health Data Space (EHDS) aims to standardize health data exchange across EU member states while maintaining strict privacy protections. *(Cross-reference Chap. 6.4 on data governance and global health policy.)*

How to Use This Workbook

The Digital Medicine Starter Guide is designed to serve as both a foundational reference and a practical toolkit for healthcare professionals endeavoring to navigate the dynamic landscape of Digital Health technologies. Unlike traditional medical textbooks that concentrate exclusively on theory, this workbook effectively bridges the divide between knowledge and application, thereby ensuring that readers are equipped to critically assess, implement, and optimize digital tools in actual clinical environments.

Throughout this guide, you will encounter structured learning pathways, interactive case studies, practical evaluation frameworks, and cross-disciplinary insights, socio-economic ones, all of which contribute to a comprehensive, hands-on approach to Digital Medicine.

A Roadmap for Different Learners

The Digital Medicine Starter Guide is meticulously crafted to address a diverse audience, encompassing clinicians, medical researchers, healthcare administrators, policymakers, sociologists, economists and innovators in Digital Health. Everyone will engage with this workbook in a manner that reflects their unique background and specific objectives. Presented below is a customized roadmap for distinct user groups:

For Clinicians Seeking Practical Implementation

Commence with Chap. 1 to attain a comprehensive understanding of the nature of Digital Medicine and its distinctions. Continue to Chap. 3 for a thorough examination of specific technologies, including telemedicine, mobile health (mHealth) applications, wearable devices, and artificial intelligence-driven tools. Consult Chap. 4 to explore optimal practices for implementation within healthcare systems, which include workflow integration, stakeholder engagement, and the management of clinical resistance.

Refer to Chap. 5 for strategies to address adoption challenges, such as data privacy concerns, interoperability hurdles, and reimbursement models.

Chapter 6 examines socio-economic aspects, emphasizing that the promise of digital transformation must be aligned with equality while maintaining an epistemological focus on the individual rather than the system.

Apply knowledge from Chap. 7 to anticipate future trends and innovations in AI, predictive analytics, and personalized medicine.

For Administrators and Healthcare Executives Focused on Digital Transformation

Begin with Chap. 2 to understand how digital tools align with healthcare system needs.

Explore Chap. 6 for dedicated insights from a sociological and economic perspective." regulatory frameworks, and patient-centric care models.

Please refer to Chap. 4 for comprehensive insights regarding the scaling of digital solutions, the assurance of interoperability, and the establishment of measurable success metrics.

Use Chap. 5 to assess barriers to adoption, including cost-benefit analysis, cybersecurity threats, and workforce training needs.

Leverage Chap. 7 for long-term strategic planning, integrating insights on AI-driven automation, digital therapeutics, and evolving policy landscapes.

For Researchers and Innovators Developing New Digital Health Solutions

Focus on Chap. 3 to explore current Digital Medicine technologies, their clinical applications, and gaps in existing solutions.

Utilize Chap. 5 to discern regulatory challenges, ethical considerations, and validation frameworks pertaining to Digital Health innovations.

Read Chap. 6 to reference a value beyond matrix perspective.

Refer to Chap. 7 to gain insights into emerging fields, such as bioelectronic medicine, augmented reality (AR) in surgery, and predictive analytics for population health.

For Policymakers and Regulatory Experts Crafting Digital Health Policies

Commence with Chap. 2 to explore the integration of Digital Medicine within the broader transformations occurring in the healthcare system. Consult Chap. 5 to acquire insights regarding privacy, compliance, and security frameworks, including GDPR, HIPAA, and the European Health Data Space (EHDS). Explore Chap. 6 for further reference to socio-economic matters and value metrics. Refer to Chap. 7 for a prospective examination of global regulatory trends, ethical AI governance, and international collaboration in Digital Health policy.

By structuring this workbook as a modular and adaptive resource, readers can customize their learning journey based on their unique needs, expertise, and professional goals.

Engaging with Case Studies and Practical Exercises

This guide transcends theoretical discussion; it is meticulously structured around real-world examples, case studies, and interactive exercises designed to reinforce learning and facilitate practical implementation.

Each chapter includes:

Case studies derived from real-world implementations, specifically illustrative examples of successful Digital Medicine projects, underscore their impact, challenges, and lessons learned. Additionally, these case studies investigate the expansion of telemedicine in rural healthcare, AI-assisted radiology diagnostics, and wearable-based chronic disease management programs *(refer to Chap. 4.7 for details)*. Furthermore, practical exercises and reflective questions are included, aimed at facilitating readers in applying concepts to their respective practices.

Example. After reading about remote patient monitoring (RPM) in Chap. 3.3, a reflection exercise guides the reader to assess how RPM could be integrated into their healthcare setting.

Frameworks for Evaluating Digital Tools

Throughout this guide, checklists and assessment models help determine whether a digital tool meets the criteria for safety, efficacy, and clinical validation.

Example. The Digital Health Assessment Framework (DHA) in Chap. 4 provides a step-by-step method for evaluating digital solutions based on usability, security, and interoperability.

By engaging with these interactive components, readers acquire knowledge and cultivate the critical thinking skills essential for evaluating, implementing, and enhancing Digital Health interventions.

Leveraging Appendices, Resources, and Quick Reference Tools

In order to enhance learning and facilitate practical application, this guide comprises a comprehensive appendix and reference section which offers:

- Summaries of key regulations and compliance frameworks (GDPR, HIPAA, FDA Digital Health policies).
- A glossary of essential terms in Digital Medicine (see Glossary Section for a thorough reference).
- Evaluation checklists and implementation blueprints for the seamless adoption of Digital Health technologies.
- Recommendations for further reading on artificial intelligence in medicine, interoperability standards, and Digital Health ethics.

Commitment to Continuous Learning

Digital Medicine represents a rapidly evolving field, necessitating that healthcare professionals engage in ongoing education and adaptation in order to remain at the forefront of innovation. This guide underscores the significance of the following concepts.

Keeping Up with Emerging Trends

Engaging in regular reviews of peer-reviewed journals, industry reports, and regulatory updates is essential. Participation in Digital Health conferences, online courses, and professional networks is highly encouraged. Collaboration across Disciplines: The field of Digital Medicine necessitates cooperation among clinicians, technologists, data scientists, and policymakers. For instance, the implementation of AI-driven diagnostics requires contributions from radiologists, software engineers, and ethics committees in order to ensure accuracy, safety, and compliance with regulatory standards.

Applying Knowledge to Real-World Practice

Encouraging pilot projects, research initiatives, and innovation hubs to test and refine digital solutions in clinical settings.

Example: A hospital may pilot an AI-based triage tool before expanding its use across departments (see Chap. 5.1.2 on overcoming clinician resistance).

By adopting a mindset of continuous learning, healthcare professionals are positioned to proactively influence the future of Digital Medicine. They can guarantee that technology augments care delivery, enhances patient outcomes, and maintains ethical integrity.

Final Thoughts on Using This Workbook

The *Digital Medicine Starter Guide v1.0* is not merely a static reference manual; it serves as a dynamic, interactive tool that evolves in conjunction with your professional development and the broader Digital Health ecosystem.

Whether one is a clinician implementing AI-driven diagnostics, an administrator designing telehealth strategies, a researcher developing the next breakthrough in biosensors, or a policymaker shaping regulatory frameworks, this guide provides the knowledge and practical resources essential for the effective integration of Digital Medicine into contemporary healthcare.

By the end of this guide, readers will have developed:

A comprehensive understanding of the fundamental principles, technologies, and practical applications of Digital Medicine.

A framework for the critical assessment of digital tools, ensuring clinical validation, and optimizing patient-centered care.

The confidence to embrace and lead Digital Health innovations within their organizations.

As we advance, we shall investigate how these concepts manifest into concrete healthcare solutions. Chapter 2 will commence by closely examining the foundational principles of Digital Medicine.

Suggested Reading

1. Digital Medicine Society (DiMe). "Defining Digital Medicine." Digital Medicine Society. (n.d.). Defining Digital Medicine. Retrieved from https://dimesociety.org/about-us/defining-digital-medicine/
2. U.S. Food and Drug Administration (FDA). "What is Digital Health?" U.S. Food and Drug Administration. (n.d.). What is Digital Health? Retrieved from https://www.fda.gov/medical-devices/digital-health-center-excellence/what-digital-health
3. Nature Medicine. Digital Medicine, on its way to being just plain medicine. npj Digital Med. 2018;1:20175. https://doi.org/10.1038/s41746-017-0005-1.
4. National Center for Biotechnology Information (NCBI). Applications of digital medicine in oncology: prospects and challenges. Cancer Innov. 2023;1(4):285–92. https://doi.org/10.1002/cai2.37.eCollection.
5. Digital Medicine Society (DiMe). Evidence DEFINED. n.d.. Retrieved from https://dimesociety.org/access-resources/evidence-defined/
6. The Medical Futurist. These are the top examples of digital therapeutics. 2022. Retrieved from https://medicalfuturist.com/the-new-buzz-these-are-the-top-examples-of-digital-therapeutics/
7. Talking HealthTech. Digital health, digital medicine, and digital therapeutics; what is the difference? 2021. Retrieved from https://www.talkinghealthtech.com/glossary/digital-health-digital-medicine-and-digital-therapeutics-what-is-the-difference
8. World Health Organization (WHO). Digital health. n.d.. Retrieved from https://www.who.int/health-topics/digital-health
9. Topol E. The patient will see you now: the future of Medicine is in your hands. New York: Basic Books; 2015.
10. Wang F, Casalino LP, Khullar D. Deep learning in medicine—promise, progress, and challenges. JAMA Intern Med. 2019;179(3):293–4. https://doi.org/10.1001/jamainternmed.2018.7117.
11. Steinhubl SR, Muse ED, Topol EJ. The emerging field of mobile health. Sci Transl Med. 2015;7(283):283rv3. https://doi.org/10.1126/scitranslmed.aaa3487.
12. Kvedar J, Coye MJ, Everett W. Connected health: a review of technologies and strategies to improve patient care with telemedicine and telehealth. Health Aff. 2014;33(2):194–9. https://doi.org/10.1377/hlthaff.2013.0992.
13. Cesario A, et al. Personalised Medicine meets artificial intelligence: beyond the hype towards the Metaverse. Springer; 2023.
14. Meskó B, Drobni Z, Bényei É, Gergely B, Győrffy Z. Digital health is a cultural transformation of traditional healthcare. mHealth. 2017;3:38. https://doi.org/10.21037/mhealth.2017.08.07.

15. Yu KH, Beam AL, Kohane IS. Artificial intelligence in healthcare. Nat Biomed Eng. 2018;2(10):719–31. https://doi.org/10.1038/s41551-018-0305-z.
16. Dorsey ER, Topol EJ. State of telehealth. N Engl J Med. 2016;375(2):154–61. https://doi.org/10.1056/NEJMra1601705.
17. Daniel H, Snyder Sulmasy L, Health and Public Policy Committee of the American College of Physicians. Policy recommendations to guide the use of telemedicine in primary care settings: an American College of Physicians position paper. Ann Intern Med. 2015;163(10):787–9. https://doi.org/10.7326/M15-0498.
18. Frederix I, Caiani EG, Dendale P, et al. ESC e-cardiology working group position paper: overcoming challenges in digital health implementation in cardiovascular medicine. Eur J Prev Cardiol. 2019;26(11):1166–77. https://doi.org/10.1177/2047487319832394.
19. Wang C, Lee C, Shin H. Digital therapeutics from bench to bedside. NPJ Digit Med. 2023;6:38. https://doi.org/10.1038/s41746-023-00777-z.
20. Crisafulli S, Santoro E, Recchia G, Trifirò G. Digital therapeutics in perspective: from regulatory challenges to post-marketing surveillance. Front Drug Saf Regul. 2022;2:900946. https://doi.org/10.3389/fdsfr.2022.900946.
21. Lu L, Zhang J, Xie Y, et al. Wearable health devices in health care: narrative systematic review. JMIR Mhealth Uhealth. 2020;8(11):e18907. https://doi.org/10.2196/18907.
22. Torab-Miandoab A, Samad-Soltani T, Jodati A, Rezaei-Hachesu P. Interoperability of heterogeneous health information systems: a systematic literature review. BMC Med Inform Decis Mak. 2023;23(1):18. https://doi.org/10.1186/s12911-023-02115-5.
23. Norman CD, Skinner HA. eHealth literacy: essential skills for consumer health in a networked world. J Med Internet Res. 2006;8(2):e9. https://doi.org/10.2196/jmir.8.2.e9.
24. World Health Organization. mHealth: new horizons for health through mobile technologies. Geneva: WHO; 2011. Available from: https://apps.who.int/iris/handle/10665/44607
25. World Health Organization. WHO guideline: recommendations on digital interventions for health system strengthening. Geneva: WHO; 2019. Available from: https://apps.who.int/iris/handle/10665/311941
26. World Health Organization. Global strategy on digital health 2020–2025. Geneva: WHO; 2021. Available from: https://apps.who.int/iris/handle/10665/344249
27. World Health Organization. Ethics and governance of artificial intelligence for health: WHO guidance. Geneva: WHO; 2021. Available from: https://apps.who.int/iris/handle/10665/341996
28. U.S. Food and Drug Administration. Digital health innovation action plan. Silver Spring: FDA; 2017. Available from: https://www.fda.gov/media/106331/download
29. Greaves F, Joshi I, Campbell M, et al. What is an appropriate level of evidence for a digital health intervention? Lancet. 2019;392(10165):2665–7. https://doi.org/10.1016/S0140-6736(18)33129-5.
30. Keesara S, Jonas A, Schulman K. Covid-19 and health care's digital revolution. N Engl J Med. 2020;382(23):e82. https://doi.org/10.1056/NEJMp2005835.
31. Coravos A, Khozin S, Mandl KD. Developing and adopting safe and effective digital biomarkers to improve patient outcomes. NPJ Digit Med. 2019;2:14. https://doi.org/10.1038/s41746-019-0090-4.
32. Burke LE, Ma J, Azar KMJ, et al. Current science on consumer use of mobile health for cardiovascular disease prevention: a scientific statement from the American Heart Association. Circulation. 2015;132(12):1157–213. https://doi.org/10.1161/CIR.0000000000000232.
33. Flodgren G, Rachas A, Farmer AJ, et al. Interactive telemedicine: effects on professional practice and health care outcomes. Cochrane Database Syst Rev. 2015;9:CD002098. https://doi.org/10.1002/14651858.CD002098.pub2.
34. Marcolino MS, Oliveira JAQ, D'Agostino M, et al. The impact of mHealth interventions: systematic review of systematic reviews. JMIR Mhealth Uhealth. 2018;6(1):e23. https://doi.org/10.2196/mhealth.8873.
35. European Commission. Communication on enabling the digital transformation of health and care in the digital single market; empowering citizens and building a healthier society.

COM(2018) 233 final, 25 Apr 2018. Brussels: European Commission; 2018. Available from: https://eur-lex.europa.eu/legal-content/EN/TXT/?uri=COM:2018:233:FIN
36. Eysenbach G. What is e-health? J Med Internet Res. 2001;3(2):E20. https://doi.org/10.2196/jmir.3.2.e20.
37. Topol E, editor. Preparing the healthcare workforce to deliver the digital future (Topol Review). NHS Health Education England; 2019. Available from: https://topol.hee.nhs.uk/wp-content/uploads/HEE-Topol-Review-2019.pdf
38. Bhavnani SP, Narula J, Sengupta PP. Mobile technology and the digitization of healthcare. Eur Heart J. 2016;37(18):1428–38. https://doi.org/10.1093/eurheartj/ehv770.
39. Gordon WJ, Landman A, Zhang H, Bates DW. Beyond validation: getting health apps into clinical practice. NPJ Digit Med. 2020;3:14. https://doi.org/10.1038/s41746-019-0212-z.
40. Kelly CJ, Karthikesalingam A, Suleyman M, Corrado G, King D. Key challenges for delivering clinical impact with artificial intelligence. BMC Med. 2019;17(1):195. https://doi.org/10.1186/s12916-019-1426-2.

2 Foundations of Digital Medicine

Key Concepts and Definitions

Digital vs. Digitized

A prevalent misconception is that Digital Medicine is synonymous with digitized healthcare. While digitization pertains to the conversion of paper-based medical records into electronic formats, Digital Medicine encompasses a far broader scope than this particular process.

Digitized healthcare seeks to enhance existing processes through the implementation of electronic documentation and data storage. The transition from paper prescriptions to electronic health records (EHRs) embodies a form of digitization, as it streamlines workflows without fundamentally altering their essence.

Digital Medicine, in contrast, leverages consistently generated data, sophisticated analytics, remote monitoring, and patient-centered tools to promote proactive, data-driven healthcare. For instance, clinicians can employ machine learning algorithms to identify early indications of heart failure through the analysis of subtle trends in a patient's vital signs. This methodology transforms clinical decision-making and facilitates more precise, personalized, and proactive healthcare.

Software as a Medical Device (SaMD)

In the continuously evolving domain of Digital Medicine, Software as a Medical Device (SaMD) has emerged as a significant force that challenges the traditional definitions of medical instruments. Historically, the notion of a medical device was associated with tangible instruments—such as pacemakers, stethoscopes, MRI scanners, and similar items. These were objects that could be held, seen, and felt, each designed to address specific physical needs. However, as technology has advanced, so too has the scope of medical innovation. Currently, SaMD redefines

A. Cesario et al., *Digital Medicine Starter Guide*,
https://doi.org/10.1007/978-3-032-01272-2_2

the concept of a medical device, transforming software into a standalone tool that is capable of diagnosing diseases, guiding treatments, and monitoring health—completely independent of any physical counterpart.

This evolution represents not merely a technical accomplishment; it signifies a transformative reimagining of healthcare delivery. By employing ubiquitous platforms such as smartphones, tablets, and cloud-based systems, Software as a Medical Device (SaMD) seamlessly integrates into daily life, effectively dismantling barriers between patients and healthcare providers. Consequently, with SaMD, advanced medical capabilities are no longer restricted to clinics and hospitals but are instead accessible in homes, workplaces, and even the most remote corners of the globe.

Applications of SaMD: A Revolution in Progress

The applications of Software as a Medical Device (SaMD) are as diverse as they are significant, encompassing diagnostics, therapeutic guidance, and real-time monitoring. Collectively, these applications represent a substantial advancement in our approach to health management.

Diagnostic Capabilities

One of the most significant attributes of Software as a Medical Device (SaMD) is its capability to decode intricate medical data with remarkable speed and precision. This facilitates healthcare providers in diagnosing conditions at an earlier stage and with greater accuracy, frequently utilizing tools as accessible as smartphone applications.

- *Consider a mobile application specifically designed to analyze electrocardiogram (ECG) signals. Within seconds, this application is capable of detecting potentially life-threatening arrhythmias, such as atrial fibrillation. For patients residing in remote areas, or those who may be unable to access a cardiologist in a timely manner, such a tool can represent a critical difference between life and death.*
- *Another exemplary instance of transformative technology is AI-powered imaging software. Through the analysis of medical images, including X-rays and CT scans, this technology possesses the capability to identify subtle abnormalities—such as minute lung nodules that may otherwise remain undetected. Such insights not only assist radiologists in making early diagnoses but also enhance their confidence when faced with high-stakes decisions.*

These diagnostic instruments not only augment healthcare providers' capabilities but also democratize expertise, thereby rendering advanced diagnostic resources accessible well beyond the confines of specialized facilities.

Therapeutic Guidance

In addition to identifying medical issues, Software as a Medical Device (SaMD) plays a vital role in customizing treatment plans to meet the specific needs of individual patients.

- Visualize a person with type 1 diabetes. Traditionally, calculating insulin doses required careful manual adjustments, which often resulted in errors. Nowadays, SaMD applications linked to continuous glucose monitors can analyze blood sugar levels in real-time and provide precise dosing recommendations. For patients, this leads to fewer complications, more stable glucose levels, and a greater sense of control over their condition.
- Mental health represents another domain in which Software as a Medical Device (SaMD) has demonstrated its transformative potential. For instance, cognitive behavioral therapy (CBT) applications offer structured and interactive programs designed to address anxiety, depression, and a range of other mental health issues. By adapting to the user's progress and requirements, these tools emulate specific aspects of traditional therapy, thereby providing accessibility to individuals who might otherwise lack adequate support.

These examples illustrate how Software as a Medical Device (SaMD) transcends its traditional role as a mere tool, evolving into an active collaborator in personalized healthcare.

Monitoring and Alerts

Continuous monitoring has become a fundamental aspect of contemporary medicine, while software as a medical device (SaMD) has further advanced this concept. By facilitating real-time tracking of patient data, SaMD not only identifies abnormalities but also ensures prompt intervention.

- Envision a software platform developed to monitor oxygen saturation levels in patients recovering at home from COVID-19. The identification of subtle declines in oxygen levels can serve to alert healthcare providers prior to any deterioration in the patient's condition, thereby potentially averting the need for hospitalization.
- An additional compelling illustration is the use of wearable technology, which encompasses Software as a Medical Device (SaMD) solutions. These devices are capable of monitoring various parameters, including heart rate, activity levels, and sleep patterns, thereby offering patients and healthcare providers a comprehensive perspective on health over time.

With these capabilities, Software as a Medical Device (SaMD) transforms healthcare from a reactive model—addressing issues as they arise—to a proactive approach, wherein early warnings trigger prompt actions.

The Broader Impact of SaMD: Empowering Patients and Providers

The potential of Software as a Medical Device (SaMD) extends significantly beyond its immediate medical applications. By capitalizing on the widespread availability of smartphones and other ubiquitous devices, SaMD has facilitated unprecedented access to advanced healthcare tools. This democratization of care is particularly vital for underserved communities, where the existing physical healthcare infrastructure may be insufficient, while digital tools can effectively bridge this gap.

For patients, Software as a Medical Device (SaMD) signifies empowerment. It transforms individuals from passive recipients of care into active participants, providing them with the necessary tools and insights to manage their own health effectively. For clinicians, it serves as a valuable ally, augmenting decision-making with data-driven insights that would be unattainable through manual means.

However, the impact of Software as a Medical Device (SaMD) transcends individual patients or providers. At a systemic level, its scalability—facilitated by cloud-based platforms—empowers healthcare systems to meet the demands of growing populations without overtaxing resources. This scalability guarantees that high-quality care can be delivered to a larger number of individuals more efficiently and at a diminished cost.

Navigating Challenges: Regulation and Safety

Despite the revolutionary potential of Software as a Medical Device (SaMD), its rapid evolution has prompted critical inquiries concerning safety, efficacy, and regulatory compliance. Regulatory agencies, including the Food and Drug Administration (FDA) and the Medical Device Regulation (MDR), have assiduously sought to update their frameworks, thereby guaranteeing that SaMD tools adhere to the same stringent standards as traditional medical devices. Nonetheless, as technological advancements continue to unfold, the associated challenges also evolve.

One of the most pressing issues is the proliferation of "adaptive AI," wherein algorithms learn and enhance their performance post-deployment. Although this capability possesses significant potential—providing tools that become progressively more intelligent and effective over time—it concurrently introduces substantial risks. Consequently, regulators are now assigned the responsibility of identifying methods to harmonize innovation with accountability, ensuring that these adaptive systems remain secure and dependable as they develop.

The Future of SaMD: Endless Possibilities

As Software as a Medical Device (SaMD) continues to advance, its potential appears boundless. It signifies not merely a technological innovation but also a philosophical transformation in our approach to healthcare. Where the emphasis once resided on addressing diseases post-emergence, SaMD paves the way for a future in which prevention, personalization, and early intervention become the norm.

The journey of Software as a Medical Device (SaMD) is far from complete. With every new advancement, it expands the limits of what is achievable, providing insight into a future characterized by enhanced accessibility, efficiency, and patient-centric care. In this emerging era, SaMD transcends its role as a mere tool; it serves as a bridge that connects the potential of technology with the potential of clinical effectiveness.

Interoperability and Data Standards

As the landscape of Digital Medicine continues to expand, the necessity for seamless communication among diverse systems has become paramount. This capability to share, interpret, and utilize data effortlessly—commonly referred to as interoperability—serves as the foundation of a connected healthcare ecosystem. In its absence, even the most advanced digital tools may prove insufficient, limited to isolated systems that hinder their full potential.

Interoperability ensures the unobstructed transmission of patient data throughout the healthcare continuum, extending from primary care practitioners to specialists, hospitals, and even wearable devices. By dismantling barriers and promoting collaboration, it creates a framework for coordinated, efficient, and patient-centered care.

The Consequences of Fragmentation

In the absence of interoperability, the healthcare system often experiences inefficiencies and deficiencies that can substantially influence patient outcomes.

- Redundant Testing: When systems are isolated, healthcare providers may unintentionally repeat diagnostic tests, wasting time and resources, and potentially causing unnecessary stress for patients.
- Delayed Care: Critical clinical decisions are contingent upon real-time access to data. When information is restricted within isolated systems, delays may occur, thereby jeopardizing patient safety.
- Fragmented Patient Journeys: In the absence of a comprehensive understanding of a patient's medical history, healthcare providers may inadvertently overlook critical details, thereby leading to suboptimal or incomplete care strategies.

These challenges underscore that interoperability is not merely a technical necessity, but an essential component of delivering high-quality healthcare.

The Role of Data Standards: Building a Common Language

Achieving interoperability necessitates more than mere goodwill; it requires a unified framework that facilitates effective communication among diverse systems. This is where data standards become essential, establishing a common language for the exchange of health information. Two pivotal standards have emerged as foundational elements of this initiative:

HL7 FHIR (Fast Healthcare Interoperability Resources)

HL7 FHIR has fundamentally transformed the manner in which data is exchanged between systems. Conceived with contemporary technologies in mind, it facilitates seamless communication among electronic health records (EHRs), wearable devices, mobile applications, and various other digital instruments. By employing standardized Application Programming Interfaces (APIs), HL7 FHIR streamlines data exchange, rendering it more swift and accessible. For instance, a patient's blood pressure readings obtained from a wearable device can now be integrated directly into a hospital's EHR system, thereby providing clinicians with a real-time, comprehensive overview of the patient's health.

SNOMED CT (Systematized Nomenclature of Medicine: Clinical Terms)
In the healthcare sector, precision is of utmost importance. The Systematized Nomenclature of Medicine Clinical Terms (SNOMED CT) provides a standardized vocabulary for medical terminology, ensuring that diagnoses, treatments, and procedures are comprehensively understood across various platforms. Regardless of whether a physician in Europe documents a diagnosis as "hypertension" or a counterpart in Asia utilizes a corresponding local term, SNOMED CT guarantees that both entries are recognized as denoting the same condition. This standardization eliminates ambiguity and improves the quality of data sharing.

The Benefits of Interoperability: A Connected Future

When systems function cohesively, the advantages disseminate throughout the healthcare ecosystem, benefiting providers, patients, and administrators alike.

Enhanced Efficiency: Interoperability reduces administrative burdens by streamlining workflows. Activities such as accessing patient records and transferring data between systems become more expedient and require less labor, thus enabling clinicians to conserve valuable time.

Enhanced Patient Safety: Real-time data sharing facilitates expedited responses to critical situations. For example, an integrated alert system can inform a cardiologist of concerning trends in a patient's vital signs, thereby enabling timely interventions.

Tailored Interventions: Consolidating data from diverse sources affords a more comprehensive understanding of a patient's health. This enables the development of personalized care strategies that directly address the individual's specific needs, consequently enhancing outcomes and patient satisfaction.

Overcoming Barriers: Collaboration as the Key

While the benefits of interoperability are clearly apparent, implementing them on a substantial scale poses significant challenges. Legacy systems, proprietary technologies, and varying regional regulations often impede genuine integration. Overcoming these barriers necessitates cooperation across sectors, wherein stakeholders—including healthcare providers, technology developers, policymakers, and patients—collaborate to advance open standards and shared goals.

By prioritizing interoperability, the healthcare ecosystem can transition from fragmented systems to a cohesive and connected network. This transformation enhances the effectiveness of Digital Medicine and reinforces the fundamental promise of healthcare itself: to provide timely, safe, and patient-centered care.

Remote Patient Monitoring (RPM)

In the evolving field of Digital Medicine, remote patient monitoring (RPM) has emerged as a revolutionary method for managing patient care. By utilizing connected devices, sensors, and digital tools, RPM facilitates the continuous observation of health data outside conventional healthcare environments. This may encompass devices ranging from basic at-home blood pressure monitors connected to smartphone applications to advanced patches that ensure uninterrupted monitoring of cardiac rhythms.

RPM also incorporates Patient-Reported Outcomes (PROs)—data provided directly by patients regarding their symptoms, emotions, or responses to validated health questionnaires. These contributions add a valuable layer of subjective context to the objective data collected by devices, thereby creating a more comprehensive picture of the patient's condition. Collectively, these elements establish RPM as a cornerstone of contemporary, patient-centered care. A comprehensive risk analysis is discussed in Chap. 6.

Challenges and Considerations

Notwithstanding its transformative potential, the extensive implementation of remote patient monitoring (RPM) poses considerable challenges that necessitate strategic planning and cooperation among diverse stakeholders to effectively address. Such challenges encompass technical, logistical, and societal dimensions.

Data Overload and Interpretation

Continuous monitoring generates substantial amounts of data, which can rapidly become overwhelming for clinicians if not managed effectively. In the absence of robust analytics and filtering systems, the sheer volume of data may result in missed insights or delayed responses. To address this issue, artificial intelligence-powered algorithms are being developed to distill raw data into actionable insights, emphasizing only critical deviations and trends that necessitate attention. Nevertheless, these systems must maintain a balance between automation and human oversight to ensure that vital nuances in patient data are not overlooked.

Interoperability Issues

Numerous remote patient monitoring (RPM) devices and systems operate independently, lacking the capability to integrate seamlessly with electronic health records (EHRs) or other healthcare platforms. This fragmentation diminishes the potential of RPM by establishing obstacles to data sharing and care coordination. Standardized protocols, such as HL7 FHIR, are crucial for resolving these challenges; however, attaining true interoperability continues to be an ongoing endeavor that necessitates collaboration among technology providers, regulators, and healthcare organizations.

Digital Divide and Equity

Access to remote patient monitoring (RPM) technologies is not uniformly distributed. Rural and underserved populations may experience a deficiency in the requisite infrastructure, such as reliable Internet connectivity, hindering their ability to fully benefit from RPM solutions. Likewise, the financial implications associated with devices and subscription services can pose significant barriers for patients with lower incomes. Addressing these disparities necessitates both public and private investments in digital infrastructure, subsidies for vulnerable populations, and the development of user-friendly technologies that cater to varying levels of digital literacy.

Privacy and Security Concerns

As RPM involves the transmission and storage of sensitive health data, it is essential to ensure robust cybersecurity. Cyberattacks, data breaches, and unauthorized access present significant risks to both patients and healthcare providers. Healthcare organizations must implement stringent data protection measures, including encryption, multi-factor authentication, and secure data-sharing protocols, while complying with regulations such as GDPR and HIPAA. Educating patients about how their data is utilized and protected is equally important for nurturing trust.

Clinical Adoption and Workflow Integration

Even the most advanced remote patient monitoring (RPM) systems may face resistance from clinicians if they are perceived as burdensome or disruptive to existing workflows. Numerous healthcare providers are already overwhelmed by administrative tasks, and the introduction of new technologies without adequate training and support can further exacerbate this issue. For RPM to achieve success, it must be seamlessly integrated into clinical workflows, backed by comprehensive training programs, and user-friendly interfaces.

Regulatory and Ethical Considerations

As remote patient monitoring (RPM) technologies evolve at a rapid pace, regulatory frameworks are encountering challenges in keeping up. Issues surrounding liability, patient consent, and data ownership significantly complicate the adoption of these technologies. For example, determining liability in the event that an RPM system fails to identify a critical issue raises pertinent questions. Additionally, ethical concerns emerge regarding the risk of excessive monitoring, which could lead to unwarranted interventions or heightened anxiety for patients. Therefore, the establishment of clear and updated regulatory guidelines, in conjunction with robust ethical standards, is imperative to address these challenges and foster a safe, transparent environment for RPM.

The Future of RPM: Toward a More Connected Healthcare System

As remote patient monitoring (RPM) continues to evolve, its potential to transform healthcare delivery is significantly increasing. Innovations in device miniaturization, sensor technology, and artificial intelligence-powered analytics are enhancing the accuracy, user-friendliness, and accessibility of monitoring tools. Moreover, the integration of RPM with other Digital Health technologies—such as telemedicine platforms and electronic health records (EHRs)—is cultivating a more interconnected and efficient healthcare ecosystem.

Ultimately, remote patient monitoring (RPM) signifies a paradigm shift in the provision of healthcare services. By transcending the limitations of traditional hospital settings and incorporating itself into the daily lives of patients, it facilitates a transformation of healthcare from a reactive model to one that is proactive, personalized, and profoundly empowering. In this innovative context, the patient is not simply a recipient of care, but rather an active participant, bolstered by technology that harmonizes healthcare with their unique needs and lifestyle.

Overview of Digital Tools in Medicine

Telemedicine and Telehealth

In the realm of digital healthcare transformation, *telemedicine* and *telehealth* stand out as crucial innovations that are changing the way care is delivered and accessed. While these terms are often used interchangeably, they represent distinct but complementary areas. *Telemedicine* specifically refers to the delivery of remote clinical services like virtual consultations, diagnoses, and follow-ups, allowing for direct digital interactions between patients and healthcare providers. On the other hand, *telehealth* encompasses a broader scope that includes not only clinical care but also provider training, administrative meetings, remote patient education, and public health initiatives. Together, they form a comprehensive framework for delivering healthcare remotely.

The advantages of telemedicine and telehealth are numerous. Patients benefit from unparalleled convenience by receiving care from the comfort of their homes, eliminating the need for travel or enduring lengthy waits in crowded clinics. This is particularly beneficial for individuals with mobility challenges, chronic conditions, or those residing in remote or underserved areas. Concurrently, healthcare providers can extend their services to populations that may otherwise encounter barriers to care, thus contributing to the bridging of gaps in accessibility and equity.

Transforming the Patient Experience

Consider a patient with a chronic condition, like asthma. In the past, managing flare-ups often required frequent visits to a clinic. Nowadays, a telemedicine consultation enables the patient to connect with a specialist via video call, discuss symptoms, and adjust their treatment plan—all from the comfort of home. This convenience not only enhances the patient's experience but also reduces the pressure on healthcare infrastructure.

In addition to personalized care, telehealth facilitates broader initiatives, such as virtual training sessions for healthcare providers in rural areas and community education programs on topics such as vaccine awareness. These applications exemplify telehealth's capacity to transform healthcare delivery at both micro and macro levels.

Challenges and Future Directions

Despite the evident advantages, the widespread implementation of telemedicine and telehealth introduces its own set of challenges. Ensuring equitable access continues to be a priority, given that reliable internet connectivity and digital literacy differ across various regions and demographics. Furthermore, the integration of telehealth platforms with existing electronic health record (EHR) systems, along with compliance to privacy regulations such as HIPAA and GDPR, is vital for the effective scaling of these solutions. Nevertheless, as technology progresses and public acceptance increases, telemedicine and telehealth are positioned to become fundamental components of contemporary healthcare.

Wearables and Biosensors

The emergence of *wearable technology* and *biosensors* has fundamentally transformed health monitoring and management. These devices, encompassing wrist-worn smartwatches and implantable sensors, furnish real-time insights into physiological data for both patients and clinicians. They facilitate the continuous monitoring of essential health metrics, thereby bridging the gap between intermittent clinical assessments and daily life.

Examples of Cutting-Edge Devices

Smartwatches with ECG Capabilities

Devices equipped with electrocardiogram (ECG) capabilities, such as smartwatches, are capable of identifying atrial fibrillation, a prevalent yet frequently undiagnosed cardiac rhythm disorder. Upon detection of an irregular heartbeat, the device promptly alerts the user and transmits relevant data to their healthcare provider, thereby facilitating timely intervention and minimizing the risk of complications, including stroke.

Continuous Glucose Monitors (CGMs)

For individuals diagnosed with diabetes, continuous glucose monitors (CGMs) present a transformative solution. These devices continuously monitor blood glucose levels, offering immediate feedback as well as trend analyses. Users are empowered to make informed decisions concerning their diet, exercise, and insulin administration, thereby significantly enhancing glycaemic control.

Empowering Patients and Clinicians

Wearables and biosensors serve a purpose beyond merely monitoring health; they empower patients by offering actionable insights readily accessible at their fingertips. For instance, an individual utilizing a smartwatch may modify their activity levels or stress management strategies in response to heart rate variability data. Concurrently, clinicians obtain a more comprehensive understanding of their patients' health, as these devices generate substantial data that enhances traditional assessments.

Expanding Applications

The applications of wearables and biosensors extend significantly beyond these aforementioned examples. Respiratory monitors aid patients suffering from conditions such as chronic obstructive pulmonary disease (COPD), while implantable sensors facilitate the tracking of internal biomarkers to offer early warnings of infections or organ dysfunction. Additionally, emerging technologies within this domain include sweat-based biosensors for noninvasive monitoring of electrolytes and glucose, as well as wearable patches designed to administer drugs transdermally while concurrently monitoring patient responses.

Challenges and Considerations

Despite their potential, wearables and biosensors face numerous challenges. Data accuracy and reliability continue to require improvement, as readings from these devices may occasionally be influenced by factors such as motion or improper usage. Additionally, the integration of data from these devices into clinical workflows demands seamless interoperability and robust privacy safeguards. Ultimately, addressing cost barriers and ensuring accessibility is vital to mitigate disparities in adoption, particularly among underserved populations.

A Vision for the Future

As wearable technology and biosensors continue to evolve, their role in preventive care, chronic disease management, and personalized medicine is expanding significantly. By integrating these tools with artificial intelligence and machine learning, the healthcare industry is progressing toward a future wherein data-driven, patient-centered care is established as the standard. These technologies exemplify how Digital Medicine can empower individuals and improve healthcare delivery for the greater good.

Artificial Intelligence (AI) and Machine Learning (ML)

Few technologies have captivated the imagination and transformative potential of Digital Medicine quite like Artificial Intelligence (AI) and Machine Learning (ML). These tools empower machines to analyze extensive and intricate datasets, identify patterns, and generate actionable insights, thus redefining healthcare delivery across numerous dimensions. From improving diagnostic accuracy to optimizing operational processes, AI and ML are leading a revolution intended to render healthcare more precise, predictive, and efficient.

Machine learning constitutes the most ubiquitous subset of artificial intelligence (AI). It can be defined as a collection of methodologies employed for deriving inferences and predictions from data. Prediction pertains to the anticipated outcomes of forthcoming events, whereas inference involves the extraction of insights. The methodologies associated with machine learning are primarily rooted in the disciplines of statistics and computer science. This approach is notably powerful as it empowers computers to learn autonomously, without the necessity for explicit programming. In essence, machine learning systematically identifies patterns within existing data and applies these findings to novel datasets.

At their core, artificial intelligence (AI) and machine learning (ML) function by training algorithms on extensive datasets. This process enables these technologies to "learn" from historical data and apply that knowledge to address novel challenges. As these models advance, their ability to assist clinicians, optimize processes, and even predict patient outcomes increases exponentially.

Applications of AI in Digital Medicine

Diagnostics

Artificial intelligence-powered diagnostic tools are regarded as some of the most esteemed applications of these technologies. They significantly enhance the accuracy, consistency, and speed of disease identification and frequently surpass human specialists in particular tasks.

Example: AI models analyzing imaging scans can swiftly identify abnormalities such as fractures, cancers, or neurological conditions, supplying clinicians with prompt and accurate results.

Example: Google's DeepMind AI system can identify over 50 eye conditions from retinal imaging with exceptional accuracy, frequently exceeding human ophthalmologists in both speed and precision.

Predictive Analytics

Predictive analytics utilizes AI to anticipate patient risks and enable early interventions, thereby minimizing complications and improving outcomes.

Example: Machine learning algorithms use EHR data to identify patients at high risk for conditions like sepsis, hospital readmissions, or adverse drug reactions. These predictions allow healthcare teams to implement preventive strategies, saving lives and resources.

Clinical Decision Support Systems (cDSS)

AI-driven Clinical Decision Support Systems (cDSS) provide evidence-based recommendations personalized for individual patients, enabling clinicians to make informed decisions.

Example: Oncology platforms that utilize AI offer personalized treatment plans customized to tumour genomics, clinical guidelines, and patient characteristics, aiding oncologists in navigating the complexities of cancer care.

Operational Optimization

In addition to its clinical applications, artificial intelligence significantly enhances the efficiency of healthcare systems. By automating administrative tasks, optimizing resource allocation, and improving patient interactions, artificial intelligence aids in reducing operational bottlenecks.

AI-enabled chatbots can manage patient inquiries, assist with appointment scheduling, and offer basic health advice, allowing administrative staff to focus on more complex responsibilities.

Digital Twins: Simulating Healthcare in a Virtual World

One of the most innovative applications of artificial intelligence in the field of Digital Medicine is the development of Digital Twins. A Digital Twin is defined as a virtual replica of a physical entity—specifically, a patient—that assimilates real-world data from diverse sources to model, simulate, and forecast health outcomes. Through the integration of data from electronic health records (EHRs), wearable devices, biosensors, and imaging studies, Digital Twins offer a comprehensive and dynamic representation of an individual's health status.

How Digital Twins Work

Digital Twins function by aggregating both real-time and historical patient data into a comprehensive model. This virtual replica develops concurrently with the patient, integrating updates from new tests, treatments, and daily health metrics. Sophisticated AI algorithms scrutinize the twin to simulate disease progression, assess treatment alternatives, and forecast outcomes, thereby allowing clinicians to investigate "what if" scenarios without posing any risk to the patient.

Applications of Digital Twins in Healthcare

Personalized Medicine: Digital Twins can simulate the potential responses of a patient to various medications, thereby assisting clinicians in the selection of the most effective treatment while minimizing side effects. For instance, in the field of oncology, a Digital Twin can predict how a tumor may react to different therapies, facilitating precise interventions.

Surgical Planning: Digital Twins provide a virtual rehearsal environment for complex surgical procedures. Surgeons are able to refine their techniques, anticipate potential challenges, and improve their strategies prior to entering the operating room.

Chronic Disease Management: Digital twins facilitate ongoing monitoring and simulation of chronic conditions, such as heart disease and diabetes. By modeling the effects of lifestyle modifications or pharmacological interventions, these technologies empower both patients and healthcare providers to make well-informed decisions.

Population Health: In addition to the care provided to individuals, Digital Twins have the capability to represent entire populations. This advancement allows researchers and policymakers to simulate public health scenarios, including the dissemination of infectious diseases and the effects of health interventions on extensive health outcomes.

Benefits and Future Potential

The strength of Digital Twins lies in their ability to amalgamate precision with predictive capabilities. By simulating the intricacies of individual health, they diminish the reliance on trial-and-error methodologies, expedite treatment timelines, and enhance patient safety. As technology progresses, the incorporation of artificial intelligence, large datasets, and advanced simulation tools is poised to reveal new opportunities, thereby positioning Digital Twins as a pivotal component of forthcoming healthcare innovation.

Opportunities and Challenges

The potential of artificial intelligence in digital medicine is considerable. It provides opportunities to transform the delivery, experience, and management of healthcare. Nevertheless, these opportunities also pose unique challenges that necessitate careful consideration.

Opportunities

Efficiency: By automating repetitive tasks, such as data entry and image analysis, artificial intelligence decreases clinician burnout and administrative expenses, thereby enabling healthcare providers to concentrate more on patient care.

Scalability: Artificial Intelligence systems possess the capability to process and analyze data at speeds and scales that are unparalleled by human efforts, thereby facilitating a more comprehensive approach to population health management.

Personalization: Algorithms developed using patient-specific data have the capacity to tailor interventions to fulfill individual requirements, consequently improving the quality and precision of care.

Challenges

Algorithmic Bias: Artificial intelligence models are significantly dependent on the data utilized for their training. In instances where the datasets exhibit a lack of diversity, AI systems may inadvertently perpetuate existing health disparities, thereby disproportionately impacting marginalized communities.

Regulatory Oversight: Comprehensive regulatory frameworks are vital for guaranteeing the safety, effectiveness, and ethical application of artificial intelligence systems, particularly those possessing adaptive or self-learning capabilities. The challenge resides in the development and continual updating of these frameworks to maintain alignment with the swift pace of innovation.

Explainability: In order for clinicians and patients to trust the recommendations made by AI tools, it is essential that they understand the rationale underlying these recommendations. Enhancing the transparency and interpretability of AI decision-making processes is crucial for fostering broader acceptance.

A Vision for the Future

The integration of artificial intelligence (AI) and machine learning (ML) into Digital Medicine signifies a paradigm shift that transcends technological advancement; it challenges and redefines the boundaries of what can be achieved in the healthcare sector. From the prevention of diseases before their onset to the personalization of treatments at the genetic level, AI is steering the medical field toward a more proactive, inclusive, and data-driven future.

Nonetheless, realizing this vision necessitates a balanced approach—one that embraces innovation while addressing its ethical, technical, and societal implications. Through sustained collaboration among clinicians, technologists, regulators, and patients, artificial intelligence has the potential to transform healthcare and enhance the core of the human experience.

Mobile Health (mHealth) Applications

The emergence of mobile health (mHealth) applications signifies one of the most transformative elements of Digital Medicine. These smartphone-based tools extend healthcare beyond traditional clinical environments, empowering users to monitor, manage, and enhance their health in real-time. Ranging from chronic disease management to support for mental health, mHealth applications are redefining patient engagement, promoting self-management, and integrating digital resources into everyday life.

Empowering Patients Through Personalized Care

In contrast to conventional healthcare models that depend on sporadic clinical interactions, mobile health (mHealth) applications present a paradigm wherein patients maintain continuous connectivity with their healthcare providers. These applications facilitate users in documenting symptoms, monitoring physiological indicators, receiving instantaneous feedback, and engaging with virtual coaching systems.

For example, a diabetes management application may integrate with a continuous glucose monitor (CGM), consolidating blood sugar data with information regarding diet, exercise, and medication adherence. Insights powered by artificial intelligence can subsequently furnish personalized recommendations, notifying users of trends that may necessitate intervention. In a similar vein, hypertension management applications can monitor blood pressure readings, providing reminders for medication adherence and informing healthcare providers of any concerning fluctuations.

Mental health represents another domain in which mHealth applications have exhibited considerable influence. Cognitive behavioral therapy (CBT) applications provide systematic, guided interventions designed to address anxiety, depression, and stress-related disorders. Several applications incorporate voice and sentiment analysis, which identifies nuanced indicators within speech patterns that signal mood fluctuations, thus enabling timely intervention.

Enhancing Clinician-Patient Collaboration

Mobile health (mHealth) applications are not exclusively focused on patients; they also function as indispensable tools for clinicians and healthcare teams. By facilitating remote patient monitoring (RPM), these applications offer real-time access to user-generated health data. This data-driven methodology empowers healthcare providers to identify early warning signs, adjust treatment plans dynamically, and participate in data-informed decision-making.

For instance, in the field of cardiology, applications that monitor heart rate variability and activity levels can facilitate the identification of episodes of atrial fibrillation, thereby prompting early interventions. In the realm of oncology, mobile health platforms empower patients undergoing chemotherapy to report side effects, consequently enabling oncologists to optimize real-time symptom management. These applications foster a continuous loop of care, which reduces unnecessary hospital visits and enhances clinical outcomes.

Integration with Broader Digital Health Ecosystems

One of the most significant strengths of mHealth is its capacity to integrate seamlessly with other Digital Health technologies. Progressively, these applications are interconnected with:

Wearables and biosensors (e.g., Apple Watch, Fitbit, Oura Ring) for real-time tracking.

Electronic Health Records (EHRs) to provide clinicians with patient-generated health data.

AI-driven clinical decision support systems (CDSS), enabling predictive analytics for more proactive care.

A well-integrated mHealth ecosystem ensures that patients' data is not siloed but rather contributes meaningfully to their broader healthcare journey.

Challenges and Considerations in mHealth Adoption

Although it holds significant promise, the widespread adoption of mHealth applications entails several challenges that need to be addressed.

Regulatory Oversight and Evidence-Based Validation

In contrast to conventional medical practices, numerous mobile health applications (mHealth) are launched into the market without undergoing stringent clinical validation. Regulatory authorities, including the Food and Drug Administration (FDA) in the United States and the Medical Device Regulation (MDR) in the European Union, have initiated the classification of specific high-risk digital health applications as Software as a Medical Device (SaMD), thereby requiring regulatory approval. Nevertheless, a significant number of wellness-oriented applications continue to operate without regulation, which raises substantial concerns regarding their safety, reliability, and accuracy.

Data Privacy and Security

Considering that mHealth applications gather and retain sensitive health information, it is imperative to implement stringent data protection measures. Adherence to

GDPR (EU), HIPAA (USA), and relevant regional privacy regulations is essential to avert unauthorized access and to protect user confidentiality.

Digital Divide and Accessibility

While mobile health applications have the potential to democratize healthcare, inequities in technological access, digital literacy, and affordability may constrain their accessibility. Implementing multilingual support, designing user-friendly interfaces, and incorporating offline functionalities can significantly improve the inclusivity of these tools.

User Engagement and Long-Term Adherence

Although initial engagement with mHealth applications tends to be high, sustained usage typically declines over time. The implementation of gamification strategies, including achievement badges, interactive coaching, and AI-driven personalization, can effectively motivate users to maintain their engagement.

The Future of mHealth Applications

As advancements in artificial intelligence (AI) and machine learning (ML) persist, mobile health (mHealth) applications are expected to evolve into more intelligent and proactive companions. Future innovations may include predictive health insights, digital twins for personal health modeling, and augmented reality (AR)-based patient education tools.

By seamlessly integrating real-time monitoring, clinical decision support, and patient engagement, mHealth applications will assume a pivotal role in preventive, participatory, and personalized healthcare—bringing Digital Medicine directly into the hands of patients.

Ethical and Regulatory Considerations

Privacy and Data Security

With the proliferation of digital tools, the safeguarding of patient data is of utmost importance. Frameworks such as the General Data Protection Regulation (GDPR) and the Health Insurance Portability and Accountability Act (HIPAA) provide comprehensive guidelines for the secure collection, storage, and sharing of health data. Ensuring compliance with these frameworks is essential for maintaining public trust.

Informed Consent in the Digital Age

In the realm of Digital Medicine, informed consent transcends conventional forms. It is imperative that patients comprehend the methods by which their data will be collected, utilized, and disseminated, as well as any potential risks associated with

AI-powered tools. Ongoing communication and transparency are crucial for fostering trust and ensuring ethical practices.

Addressing Bias and Health Equity

Algorithmic bias in artificial intelligence systems has the potential to perpetuate health disparities, particularly among underrepresented populations. To promote inclusivity, developers must prioritize the utilization of diverse training datasets and comprehensive validation processes. Additionally, policymakers and organizations must strive to mitigate digital divides by enhancing access to technology within underserved communities.

Value Assessment and Evidence Generation

In order to facilitate widespread adoption, Digital Medicine tools must unequivocally demonstrate their value through comprehensive evaluation. This encompasses:

Clinical Effectiveness: Proven improvements in patient outcomes.
Economic Feasibility: Cost savings for healthcare systems.
Real-World Evidence: Post-market surveillance to assess performance in diverse settings.

Frameworks such as the European Union's Health Technology Assessment Regulation facilitate the systematic evaluation of novel technologies, thereby guaranteeing prompt access to innovations.

Beyond Technology: The Cultural Shift

The success of Digital Medicine does not rely exclusively on technological innovation; it demands a substantial cultural transformation within healthcare systems, professional mindsets, and patient expectations. The transition from traditional, episodic healthcare models to continuous, data-driven care obliges stakeholders—clinicians, patients, administrators, and policymakers—to reevaluate how healthcare is provided, experienced, and valued.

Reimagining the Clinician's Role in a Digital World

The integration of digital tools into clinical practice represents not merely an enhancement; rather, it constitutes a fundamental shift in the manner in which healthcare providers engage with patients. Clinicians are required to transition from being solitary decision-makers to assuming the role of interpreters of intricate digital insights, thereby balancing clinical expertise with data-driven recommendations.

For instance, AI-powered decision support systems assist radiologists in identifying anomalies within imaging procedures; however, the presence of human oversight continues to be imperative. Additionally, wearable devices and biosensors generate extensive streams of patient data, thereby imposing challenges on clinicians in the realms of data interpretation and personalized recommendations. Furthermore, telemedicine significantly transforms patient interactions, necessitating the acquisition of new competencies in virtual communication and digital empathy.

Medical education and professional training must progress to equip healthcare professionals with the necessary competencies to effectively integrate digital tools. Digital literacy, ethics in artificial intelligence, and the design of human-centered technology should be incorporated as core components of clinical curricula and ongoing professional development.

Bridging the Gap Between Technology and Patient Trust

Patients must place their trust in Digital Health innovations to fully adopt and benefit from the advantages these technologies provide. Nonetheless, a considerable number of individuals persist in expressing skepticism concerning data privacy, artificial intelligence-driven diagnoses, and remote monitoring practices. To cultivate trust, healthcare organizations must prioritize the following facets:

(a) Transparency in how data is collected, used, and shared.
(b) User-friendly experiences that ensure accessibility across diverse populations.
(c) Clear communication on the benefits and limitations of digital tools.

For example, a patient utilizing a wearable ECG monitor should comprehend its clinical significance rather than simply receiving raw data points. Similarly, AI-powered chatbots should be designed with compassionate, human-centered communication styles to enhance patient engagement rather than substitute human interactions.

Fostering a Collaborative, Interdisciplinary Approach

Digital medicine thrives within collaborative ecosystems where clinicians, technologists, data scientists, policymakers, and patients engage collectively. The healthcare sector must dismantle traditional silos and foster cross-disciplinary partnerships to cultivate patient-centered, ethically robust digital innovations.

Public-private partnerships can enhance accessibility to Digital Health through investments in infrastructure. Regulatory bodies must collaborate with technology developers to establish clear and adaptable governance frameworks. Furthermore, patient advocacy groups should assume an active role in shaping the design and evaluation of digital tools.

Preparing for the Future of Digital Medicine

To ensure equitable and sustainable digital transformation, healthcare organizations must:

(a) Emphasize Digital Literacy—Train clinicians, administrators, and patients to use and interpret Digital Health technologies effectively.
(b) Reimagine Workflow Integration—Align digital tools with clinical priorities to prevent exacerbating the workload burdens on healthcare professionals.
(c) Adopt an Iterative, Learning-Based Approach—Implement pilot programs, gather real-world evidence, and refine digital strategies based on continuous feedback.

By cultivating a culture of adaptability, collaboration, and ethical responsibility, the healthcare ecosystem can realize the full potential of Digital Medicine. This approach will guarantee that innovation is not only technically impressive but also clinically meaningful, equitable, and centered on human needs.

Case Studies and Practical Exercises

Case Studies

Case Study: IDx-DR—AI-Driven Diabetic Retinopathy Screening

Summary: IDx-DR is an FDA-approved artificial intelligence software that autonomously detects diabetic retinopathy from retinal images. This software as a medical device (SaMD) facilitates earlier diagnosis in primary care settings, thereby alleviating the burden on ophthalmologists and enhancing access to care.
Key Takeaways: Regulatory approval, clinical validation, AI transparency.

Case Study: The UK NHS Digital Interoperability Initiative

Summary: The National Health Service (NHS) of the United Kingdom has successfully implemented Fast Healthcare Interoperability Resources (FHIR)-based interoperability to facilitate the connection of Electronic Health Record (EHR) systems across hospitals and primary care providers. This initiative ensures a seamless exchange of data and enhances the coordination of care.
Key Takeaways: Importance of standardization (HL7 FHIR), improved patient data sharing, interoperability challenges.

Case Study: RPM in Heart Failure Management (The CHAMPION Trial)

Summary: The CHAMPION study has demonstrated that the utilization of implantable pulmonary artery pressure sensors, when combined with remote monitoring tools, results in a reduction of hospitalizations for patients suffering from heart failure.

Key Takeaways: Early intervention, reduction in healthcare costs, patient empowerment.

Case Study: Teladoc—Telemedicine for Chronic Disease Management

Summary: Teladoc Health provides virtual consultations, remote monitoring, and AI-driven decision support for managing chronic diseases like diabetes and hypertension.

Key Takeaways: Scalability of telemedicine, improved patient adherence, regulatory hurdles.

Practical Exercises

Exercise #1: Evaluation of a Software as a Medical Device (SaMD) Solution
Select an actual SaMD, such as AI-driven electrocardiogram interpretation or skin cancer detection software. Conduct a meticulous analysis of its regulatory approval, clinical validation, and interoperability with healthcare systems.

Reflection Question: What are the key risks and opportunities associated with this technology?

Exercise #2: Identifying Interoperability Gaps in Healthcare
Conduct an investigation of an Electronic Health Record (EHR) system employed in your geographical area. Outline its limitations in data sharing and elucidate how Fast Healthcare Interoperability Resources (FHIR) standards could facilitate improved integration.

Reflection Question: What are the biggest barriers to achieving full interoperability?

Exercise #3: Designing a Pilot Program for Remote Monitoring
Assume that you have been assigned the responsibility of implementing remote patient monitoring (RPM) for patients undergoing post-surgical recovery. Please delineate the strategy for data collection, the criteria for device selection, and the methodology for patient engagement.

Reflection Question: How would you ensure compliance with data privacy regulations?

Suggested Reading

1. U.S. Food and Drug Administration. Software as a Medical Device (SaMD). 2022. Retrieved from https://www.fda.gov/medical-devices/digital-health-center-excellence/software-medical-device-samd.
2. European Medicines Agency. Medical Devices Regulation (MDR). 2023. Retrieved from https://www.ema.europa.eu/en/human-regulatory/overview/medical-devices.
3. Topol E. The creative destruction of medicine: how the digital revolution will create better healthcare. Basic Books; 2013.
4. Digital Therapeutics Alliance. What are digital therapeutics? n.d. Retrieved from https://dtxalliance.org.
5. Mittelstadt BD, Floridi L. The ethics of big data: current and foreseeable issues in biomedical contexts. Sci Eng Ethics. 2016;22(2):303–41. https://doi.org/10.1007/s11948-015-9652-2.
6. Steinhubl SR, Muse ED, Topol EJ. Can mobile health apps help improve patient care? JAMA. 2015;310(22):2395–6. https://doi.org/10.1001/jama.2013.281078.
7. Sittig DF, Singh H. A new socio-technical model for health IT safety. BMJ Qual Saf. 2010;19(Suppl 3):i68–74. https://doi.org/10.1136/qshc.2010.042085.
8. The Medical Futurist. Digital Twins and the promise of personalized medicine. 2022. Retrieved from https://medicalfuturist.com/digital-twin-and-the-promise-of-personalized-medicine/.
9. Digital Health and Care Alliance (DHACA). "Interoperability and data standards in digital health." 2021. Retrieved from https://dhaca.org.
10. HealthIT.gov. Fast healthcare interoperability resources (FHIR). n.d. Retrieved from https://www.healthit.gov/topic/standards-technology/standards/fhir.
11. HealthIT.gov. The role of SNOMED CT in Digital Health. 2022. Retrieved from https://www.healthit.gov.
12. Wang F, Casalino LP, Khullar D. Deep learning in medicine: promise, progress, and challenges. JAMA Intern Med. 2019;179(3):293–4. https://doi.org/10.1001/jamainternmed.2018.7117.
13. Kvedar J, Coye MJ, Everett W. Connected health: a review of technologies and strategies to improve patient care. Health Aff. 2014;33(2):194–9. https://doi.org/10.1377/hlthaff.2013.0992.
14. Cesario A, et al. Personalised medicine meets artificial intelligence: beyond the hype towards the Metaverse. Springer; 2023.
15. European Commission. Ethical guidelines for trustworthy AI. 2019. Retrieved from https://ec.europa.eu.
16. International Medical Device Regulators Forum (IMDRF). Software as a medical device (SaMD): clinical evaluation. IMDRF/SaMD WG/N41 FINAL:2017. Published 21 Sept 2017. Available from the IMDRF website.
17. Medical Device Coordination Group (MDCG). Guidance on qualification and classification of software in regulation (EU) 2017/745 – MDR and Regulation (EU) 2017/746 – IVDR (MDCG 2019–11). Brussels: European Commission; 2019. Available from: EU Publications.
18. U.S. Food and Drug Administration (FDA). Digital Health Innovation Action Plan. Silver Spring: FDA; 2017. Disponibile da: FDA website (Rapporto ufficiale).
19. U.S. Food and Drug Administration (FDA). Artificial intelligence/machine learning (AI/ML)-based software as a medical device action plan. Silver Spring: FDA; 2021. Disponibile da: FDA website (Piano d'azione).
20. U.S. Food and Drug Administration (FDA). Cybersecurity in medical devices: quality system considerations and content of premarket submissions. Guidance for industry and FDA staff. Silver Spring: FDA; 2023. Disponibile da: FDA website (Linee guida ufficiali).
21. Medical Device Coordination Group (MDCG). Guidance on Cybersecurity for Medical Devices (MDCG 2019–16 Rev.1). Brussels: European Commission; 2020. Disponibile da: EU Health Security site (Linee guida ufficiali).
22. Office of the National Coordinator for Health IT (ONC). 21st century cures act: interoperability, information blocking, and health IT certification program – final rule. Washington: US HHS; 2020. Disponibile da: Federal Register (Normativa federale).

23. Commissione Europea. Comunicazione della Commissione – Trasformazione digitale della sanità e dell'assistenza nel Mercato Unico Digitale, responsabilizzazione dei cittadini e società più sana. COM(2018) 233 final, 25 Apr 2018. Disponibile da: EUR-Lex (Comunicazione ufficiale).
24. Commissione Europea. Proposta di Regolamento del Parlamento Europeo e del Consiglio che stabilisce norme armonizzate sull'intelligenza artificiale (Atto sull'IA). COM(2021) 206 final, 21 Apr 2021. Disponibile da: EUR-Lex (Proposta legislativa).
25. Commissione Europea. Proposta di Regolamento sullo Spazio Europeo dei Dati Sanitari (European Health Data Space – EHDS). COM (2022) 197 final, 3 May 2022. Disponibile da: EUR-Lex (Proposta legislativa).
26. Unione Europea. Regolamento (UE) 2016/679 del Parlamento Europeo e del Consiglio del 27 aprile 2016 – Regolamento Generale sulla Protezione dei Dati (GDPR). OJ L119, 4.5.2016, p.1–88. Disponibile da: EUR-Lex (Normativa UE).
27. High-Level Expert Group on AI. Ethics guidelines for trustworthy artificial intelligence. Brussels: European Commission; 2019. Disponibile da: EU Digital Strategy (Linee guida etiche).
28. World Health Organization (WHO). WHO Guideline: Recommendations on Digital Health Interventions for Health System Strengthening. Geneva: WHO; 2019. Disponibile da: WHO int. (Linee guida ufficiali).
29. World Health Organization (WHO). Global strategy on digital health 2020–2025. Geneva: WHO; 2021. Disponibile da: WHO int (Rapporto strategico).
30. World Health Organization (WHO). Ethics and governance of artificial intelligence for health: WHO Guidance. Geneva: WHO; 2021. Disponibile da: WHO int. (Linee guida etiche).
31. Organisation for Economic Co-operation and Development (OECD). Recommendation of the Council on Health Data Governance. OECD Legal Instrument No. 0433; adottata il 13 Dic 2016. Disponibile da: OECD (Raccomandazione internazionale).
32. World Medical Association (WMA). WMA statement on augmented intelligence in medical care. Adottata dall'Assemblea Generale WMA, Tbilisi; 2019. Disponibile da: WMA (Posizione ufficiale).
33. Kickbusch I, Piselli D, Agrawal A, et al. The lancet and financial times commission on governing health futures 2030: growing up in a digital world. Lancet. 2021;398(10312):1727–76. https://doi.org/10.1016/S0140-6736(21)01824-9.
34. Carolan JEC, McGonigle J, Dennis A, Lorgelly P, Banerjee A. Technology-enabled, evidence-driven, and patient-centered: the way forward for regulating software as a medical device. JMIR Med Inform. 2022;10(1):e34038. https://doi.org/10.2196/34038.
35. Larson DB, Magnus DC, Lungren MP, Shah NH. Regulatory frameworks for development and evaluation of artificial intelligence–based diagnostic imaging algorithms: summary and recommendations. J Am Coll Radiol. 2021;18(4):540–54. https://doi.org/10.1016/j.jacr.2020.09.060.
36. Topol EJ. High-performance medicine: the convergence of human and artificial intelligence. Nat Med. 2019;25(1):44–56. https://doi.org/10.1038/s41591-018-0300-7.
37. Chang E, Mostafa J. The use of SNOMED CT, 2013–2020: a literature review. J Am Med Inform Assoc. 2021;28(9):2017–26. https://doi.org/10.1093/jamia/ocab084.
38. Fung KW, Xu J, Murphy SN, et al. Promoting interoperability between SNOMED CT and ICD-11: lessons learned from a pilot mapping project. J Am Med Inform Assoc. 2024;31(8):1631–7. https://doi.org/10.1093/jamia/ocae143.
39. Ayaz M, Pasha MF, Alzahrani MY, Budiarto R, Stiawan D. The fast Health interoperability resources (FHIR) standard: systematic literature review of implementations, applications, challenges and opportunities. JMIR Med Inform. 2021;9(7):e21929. https://doi.org/10.2196/21929.
40. Jacob C, Sezgin E, Sanchez-Vazquez A, Ivory C. Sociotechnical factors affecting patients' adoption of mobile health tools: systematic literature review and narrative synthesis. JMIR Mhealth Uhealth. 2022;10(5):e36284. https://doi.org/10.2196/36284.
41. Rainey D, Brown Wilson C, Bloomfield J, et al. The impact of mobile health interventions on service users' health outcomes and the role of health professionals: a systematic review of systematic reviews. BMC Digit Health. 2025;3:3. https://doi.org/10.1186/s13643-024-02624-y.

42. Frederix I, Caiani EG, Dendale P, et al. ESC e-cardiology working group position paper: overcoming challenges in digital health implementation in cardiovascular medicine. Eur J Prev Cardiol. 2019;26(11):1166–77. https://doi.org/10.1177/2047487319832394.
43. Huh KY, Oh J, Lee S, Yu KS. Clinical evaluation of digital therapeutics: present and future. Healthc Inform Res. 2022;28(3):188–97. https://doi.org/10.4258/hir.2022.28.3.188.
44. Abbadessa G, Brigo F, Clerico M, et al. Digital therapeutics in neurology. J Neurol. 2022;269(3):1209–24. https://doi.org/10.1007/s00415-021-10608-4.
45. Bracciale L, Loreti P, Bianchi G. Cybersecurity vulnerability analysis of medical devices purchased by national health services. Sci Rep. 2023;13:19509. https://doi.org/10.1038/s41598-023-45927-1.
46. Freyer O, Jahed F, Ostermann M, Rosenzweig C, Werner P, Gilbert S. Consideration of cybersecurity risks in the benefit-risk analysis of medical devices: scoping review. J Med Internet Res. 2024;26:e65528. https://doi.org/10.2196/65528.
47. Katsoulakis E, Wang Q, Wu H, et al. Digital twins for health: a scoping review. NPJ Digit Med. 2024;7(1):77. https://doi.org/10.1038/s41746-024-01073-0.
48. Ringeval M, Etindele Sosso FA, Cousineau M, Paré G. Advancing health care with digital twins: meta-review of applications and implementation challenges. J Med Internet Res. 2025;27(1):e69544. https://doi.org/10.2196/69544.
49. Unione Europea. Regolamento (UE) 2017/745 del Parlamento Europeo e del Consiglio del 5 aprile 2017 relativo ai dispositivi medici (MDR). OJ L117. 2017;5(5):1–175. Available from: EUR-Lex.
50. Bundesinstitut für Arzneimittel und Medizinprodukte (BfArM). The fast-track process for digital health applications (DiGA) according to section 139e SGB V – a guide for manufacturers, service providers and users. Bonn: BfArM; 2020. Disponibile da: BfArM (Institutional Guide DiGA).

3 Digital Tools and Applications

Telemedicine: Best Practices for Remote Care

Telemedicine has rapidly emerged as a fundamental component of Digital Healthcare, revolutionizing the delivery of healthcare services by establishing connections between patients and providers across extensive distances. This transformation has been particularly pronounced during global crises, such as the COVID-19 pandemic, which underscored the pressing necessity for innovative solutions in remote healthcare. The realm of telemedicine encompasses virtual consultations, digital triage, and remote follow-ups, thereby ensuring that patients receive prompt care without the requirement for physical visits. Furthermore, it plays a vital role in enhancing healthcare accessibility for underserved populations in rural or remote regions, where medical resources may be constrained or challenging to obtain.

At its core, telemedicine aims to enhance access, convenience, and efficiency while maintaining high standards of care. It eliminates geographical barriers, allowing patients to consult specialists regardless of their location, and mitigates logistical burdens such as travel time and related costs. Furthermore, telemedicine has demonstrated significant value in decreasing waiting times for consultations, particularly for nonurgent cases, thereby liberating in-person resources for more acute or complex medical needs.

Clinical and Operational Benefits

Telemedicine offers numerous clinical benefits. It promotes early intervention by enabling quick communication between patients and healthcare providers, often leading to better health outcomes. For instance, a patient showing respiratory infection symptoms can quickly consult a clinician, receive proper advice, and avoid unnecessary trips to the emergency department. This approach not only assists individual patients but also eases the strain on overwhelmed healthcare systems by

A. Cesario et al., *Digital Medicine Starter Guide*,
https://doi.org/10.1007/978-3-032-01272-2_3

improving resource use. Additionally, virtual care platforms allow patients to receive care from their homes, minimizing their exposure to health risks.

Operationally, telemedicine enables healthcare organizations to adapt more rapidly to evolving demands. By transitioning routine consultations to an online platform, hospitals and clinics can utilize their physical resources more efficiently. For instance, primary care providers may employ telemedicine for routine follow-ups, such as monitoring chronic conditions or managing medications, while concentrating in-person efforts on emergencies or critical cases. This hybrid model enhances the overall efficiency of healthcare delivery systems.

Technological and Regulatory Foundations

Robust technological and regulatory frameworks are essential for the efficacy of telemedicine. High-speed internet connectivity, dependable video conferencing platforms, and secure communication channels are imperative for facilitating seamless virtual consultations. Security assumes particular significance, as telemedicine platforms handle sensitive.

Nonetheless, the large-scale implementation of telemedicine presents a distinct array of challenges. Variations in state and national licensing requirements frequently complicate cross-border telemedicine practices, while disparities in reimbursement policies and insurance coverage can impede widespread adoption. Addressing these regulatory barriers necessitates coordinated efforts among policymakers, healthcare providers, and technology developers to establish standardized frameworks that facilitate the efficient delivery of virtual care.

Best Practices for Implementation

The successful integration of telemedicine into healthcare systems is contingent upon meticulous planning and execution. The selection of an appropriate platform is paramount; telemedicine systems must incorporate end-to-end encryption, user-friendly interfaces, and transparent data-handling practices to ensure both security and usability. Training for healthcare providers is equally essential, as clinicians must not only acquire proficiency in the technical dimensions of telemedicine tools but also adapt their communication styles to virtual environments. Establishing rapport with patients through a digital medium necessitates nuanced adjustments, such as maintaining eye contact with the camera and employing clear, empathetic language to cultivate a sense of connection.

A patient-centered approach is essential for the success of telemedicine. Platforms should prioritize accessibility by ensuring that features such as scheduling, payment systems, and language options are both intuitive and inclusive. Furthermore, patients with limited digital literacy or access to high-speed internet must receive assistance through simplified workflows or alternative communication channels, including phone-based consultations. Such measures ensure that telemedicine solutions are equitable and do not exacerbate healthcare disparities.

Furthermore, healthcare organizations must establish clear business models that align with their telemedicine offerings. Defining the payer—patients, insurers, employers, or governmental entities—holds paramount importance in creating financially sustainable services. In the absence of a precise understanding of who will bear the cost of care, even the most innovative telemedicine solutions face the risk of not achieving widespread adoption. Demonstrating the value of telemedicine through enhanced health outcomes, cost savings, and operational efficiency can aid in securing support from key stakeholders, ultimately facilitating broader implementation.

Telemedicine in the Broader Context of Digital Medicine

The foundational principles that support telemedicine are intimately connected with the overarching objectives of Digital Medicine, as elaborated in the preceding chapters. In a manner analogous to other digital tools, telemedicine underscores the importance of accessibility, efficiency, and patient-centered care, while simultaneously complying with rigorous safety and privacy standards. The incorporation of technologies such as artificial intelligence (AI) and wearable devices significantly enhances its potential. For example, AI-powered triage systems possess the capability to assess patient-reported symptoms prior to consultations, thus directing clinicians toward more targeted and efficient interactions. Similarly, wearable devices that continuously monitor vital signs provide clinicians with critical data during virtual consultations, thereby effectively bridging the divide between remote healthcare and in-person evaluations.

By harnessing these complementary technologies, telemedicine transitions from a standalone solution to an indispensable component of an interconnected Digital Healthcare ecosystem. It functions as a conduit between patients and providers, offering a scalable and adaptable framework for delivering care within an increasingly complex and fast-paced environment. As the field of Digital Medicine continues to advance, telemedicine will undoubtedly assume a pivotal role in shaping the future of healthcare.

Mobile Health (mHealth) Apps

Mobile health (mHealth) applications exemplify some of the most accessible and influential innovations within the domain of Digital Medicine. By leveraging the omnipresence of smartphones and tablets, mHealth applications empower individuals to assume a more proactive role in managing their health, while simultaneously equipping clinicians with tools to optimize workflows and improve patient care. These applications fulfill a diverse array of purposes, ranging from the monitoring of chronic conditions and facilitating medication adherence to providing evidence-based health education and mental health support.

The transformative potential of mobile health (mHealth) resides in its capacity to connect formal healthcare environments with the daily lives of patients. By equipping individuals with essential health tools at their fingertips, mHealth applications mitigate obstacles to care while fostering proactive health management. As referenced in Chap. 2, this possibility of democratization of healthcare is in close accordance with the principles of accessibility, patient-centeredness, and equity that form the foundation of Digital Medicine.

The Widespread Reach of mHealth

Smartphones have emerged as indispensable instruments for billions of individuals globally, presenting an unparalleled opportunity to enhance healthcare services for previously underserved populations. For instance, individuals residing in rural regions with restricted access to healthcare facilities can utilize mHealth applications to monitor their conditions, receive guidance, and even establish connections with healthcare providers for virtual consultations. Similarly, those with demanding schedules or mobility challenges can reap the benefits of the convenience and flexibility these tools afford.

Nevertheless, the reach of mHealth transcends the mere enhancement of access to healthcare services. These applications also play a pivotal role in preventive health by encouraging users to adopt healthier lifestyles through functionalities such as activity monitoring, dietary recommendations, and mindfulness exercises. For instance, an individual seeking to manage hypertension may rely on an application to track their blood pressure readings, receive personalized alerts, and obtain educational resources on sustaining a heart-healthy diet. Such instruments not only improve individual health outcomes but also bolster broader public health initiatives by promoting wellness on a larger scale.

Diverse Applications of mHealth

One of the defining strengths of mobile health (mHealth) applications is their versatility. These tools can generally be classified into three primary functional areas: condition-specific management, lifestyle and wellness, and clinical decision support.

Condition-specific applications offer a personalized approach to the management of diseases for individuals with chronic conditions, such as diabetes and asthma. For instance, a diabetes application may incorporate data from a continuous glucose monitor (CGM) to track blood sugar levels in real-time, providing users with actionable insights and reminders to adhere to their treatment plans. Similarly, asthma applications can monitor triggers and medication usage, allowing users to anticipate and manage flare-ups effectively.

Lifestyle and wellness applications advocate for healthy habits and underscore the importance of preventive care. These tools frequently incorporate step counters, nutrition trackers, and guided meditation exercises, thereby promoting a holistic approach to well-being. Their intuitive interfaces and gamified elements, including badges or challenges, make these applications particularly engaging and effective in sustaining user motivation.

On the clinical front, decision-support applications empower healthcare professionals to access essential resources conveniently, including medical guidelines, diagnostic algorithms, and drug interaction databases. For example, a physician handling a complex case may employ an application to cross-reference symptoms and laboratory results with established diagnostic criteria, thereby facilitating swifter and more precise decision-making. This incorporation of mobile health (mHealth) into clinical workflows highlights its potential as a means of improving both individual patient care and overall system efficacy.

Key Considerations for Effective Adoption

While mobile health applications provide considerable benefits, their efficacy is contingent upon careful design, thorough validation, and seamless integration within the wider healthcare ecosystem. It is essential for developers and healthcare providers to prioritize the following factors to enhance the effectiveness of these tools:

User-Centered Design

The usability of a mobile health (mHealth) application is paramount for its adoption and sustained use. Applications ought to incorporate intuitive interfaces that cater to users possessing diverse levels of digital literacy. For instance, the integration of larger fonts, voice assistance, and multilingual options can significantly enhance accessibility for older adults or non-native speakers. Furthermore, engaging features such as progress trackers or motivational notifications serve to sustain user interest and promote adherence to health objectives.

Clinical Validation

As emphasized in Chap. 2, mobile health (mHealth) tools must be rooted in evidence-based practices. This necessitates that any recommendations or features presented by the application are rigorously tested and validated by healthcare professionals. For instance, a symptom tracking application that offers diagnostic suggestions must be substantiated by reliable clinical algorithms to guarantee its accuracy and safety.

Data Security and Privacy

Considering the sensitive nature of health data, mobile health (mHealth) applications are required to comply with stringent privacy standards, including the General Data Protection Regulation (GDPR) and the Health Insurance Portability and

Accountability Act (HIPAA). Implementing encryption, anonymization, and transparent data usage policies is essential for preserving user trust. Moreover, patients should be informed about how their data will be utilized, stored, and shared, thereby ensuring their active participation in their healthcare.

Interoperability and Integration

Applications must seamlessly integrate with other digital tools and healthcare systems to realize the full potential of mobile health (mHealth). For instance, an application that monitors blood pressure readings should possess the capability to share data with electronic health records (EHRs), thereby enabling clinicians to acquire a comprehensive overview of the patient's health. Similarly, interoperability with wearable devices and biosensors facilitates the provision of richer, real-time insights.

Equity and Accessibility

Ensuring equitable access to mobile health (mHealth) applications is essential for addressing disparities in digital healthcare. Developers should consider the needs of underserved populations by offering affordable solutions that are compatible with lower-cost devices and functional in areas with limited Internet connectivity. Government subsidies, partnerships between public and private sectors, and community education initiatives can also encourage widespread adoption. These concepts will be extensively discussed in Chap. 6.

The Role of mHealth in Digital Medicine

mHealth applications exemplify the principles of Personalized, Participatory, Preventive, and Predictive (P4) Medicine outlined in Chap. 1. By combining convenience, accessibility, and clinical rigor, these tools empower patients to take charge of their health while enabling clinicians to deliver more targeted and effective care. Furthermore, mHealth acts as a vital link in the broader Digital Health ecosystem, complementing telemedicine, wearables, and artificial intelligence (AI) technologies.

For instance, a mobile health (mHealth) application designed to monitor a patient's dietary habits and physical activity could transmit data to a wearable device that records vital signs. This information would be utilized by an artificial intelligence (AI) algorithm that analyzes trends and detects potential health risks. This interconnected methodology illustrates the future of healthcare, wherein digital instruments function collaboratively to provide comprehensive, patient-centered care.

By bridging the gap between daily life and formal healthcare environments, mHealth applications improve personal health outcomes and possess the potential to significantly transform public health on a larger scale. As these tools continue to evolve, their integration into healthcare systems will be essential for realizing the full potential of Digital Medicine.

Wearables and Biosensors

Wearable devices and biosensors constitute one of the most dynamic frontiers in the realm of Digital Medicine, providing continuous, real-time insights into human physiology. These instruments extend healthcare beyond conventional clinical environments, facilitating the monitoring and management of health conditions in daily life. Ranging from fitness trackers that quantify steps and caloric intake to sophisticated medical-grade sensors capable of detecting irregular heart rhythms or monitoring glucose levels, wearables and biosensors effectively bridge the divide between episodic clinical evaluations and the ongoing reality of navigating health challenges. They exemplify the principles of personalized, preventive, and participatory care, as articulated in Chap. 1, and 2.

The Value of Continuous Monitoring

One of the defining characteristics of wearable devices and biosensors is their capacity to continuously capture and transmit physiological data. In contrast to traditional healthcare models that depend on periodic check-ups or snapshot data, these devices offer a more comprehensive perspective on a patient's health status. For example, a smartwatch incorporating an electrocardiogram (ECG) sensor is capable of monitoring heart rhythms throughout the day, thereby identifying real-time anomalies such as atrial fibrillation. This early detection facilitates timely intervention, potentially averting severe complications such as strokes.

Continuous glucose monitors (CGMs) signify a substantial advancement, particularly for individuals diagnosed with diabetes. By measuring glucose levels at regular intervals and supplying actionable feedback, CGMs empower users to modify their dietary habits, exercise regimens, or insulin dosages as necessary. This degree of precision diminishes the likelihood of hypo- or hyperglycemic episodes and significantly improves overall quality of life.

In addition to specific conditions, wearable devices also assume a significant role in preventative healthcare. Devices that monitor sleep patterns, stress levels, and physical activity provide users with actionable insights designed to enhance their overall well-being. For example, a wearable device that detects a decline in physical activity over several days may encourage users to establish new fitness goals, thereby promoting proactive health management.

Empowering Patients and Clinicians

Wearable devices and biosensors provide significant resources directly to patients, thereby empowering them to adopt a more proactive approach in managing their health. By furnishing immediate feedback, these devices assist users in making informed choices regarding their lifestyles and treatment strategies. For instance, individuals recuperating from cardiac surgery may utilize a wearable device to monitor their physical activity, thereby ensuring compliance with prescribed rehabilitation protocols while preventing overexertion.

For healthcare professionals, wearable devices afford exceptional access to extensive longitudinal datasets. These continuous streams of data can enhance diagnostic precision and inform personalized treatment strategies. In the management of chronic diseases, for instance, a biosensor that monitors blood pressure or oxygen saturation provides a comprehensive perspective on a patient's condition over time, enabling clinicians to adjust treatments proactively. The integration of wearable technology into clinical workflows aligns with the overarching objectives of Digital Medicine by optimizing care delivery and outcomes.

Expanding Applications in Healthcare

The versatility of wearables and biosensors encompasses numerous medical disciplines. In the field of cardiology, for example, smartwatches equipped with electrocardiogram (ECG) functionality are capable of detecting arrhythmias and providing patients with lifestyle recommendations aimed at enhancing cardiovascular health. In the realm of respiratory care, wearable monitors that assess lung function assist patients suffering from asthma or chronic obstructive pulmonary disease (COPD) in identifying triggers and managing symptoms more effectively.

The emergence of innovations in wearable technology continues to broaden their scope. For example, sweat-based biosensors possess the capability to noninvasively monitor hydration, electrolytes, and even glucose levels, thereby creating new opportunities for the management of conditions such as diabetes or heat-related illnesses. Furthermore, implantable biosensors present even greater potential, with applications that range from monitoring internal biomarkers to administering medications in response to detected physiological changes. These advancements underscore the evolving role of wearables and biosensors in enabling precision medicine.

Challenges and Limitations

While wearables and biosensors offer considerable advantages, the extensive adoption of these technologies faces certain challenges. The *accuracy and reliability* of data continue to be paramount concerns. Variability in sensor performance, attributable to motion artifacts, environmental influences, or improper usage, may lead to inconsistent readings, thereby undermining user trust. For example, should a fitness tracker inaccurately quantify steps or calorie expenditure, it could result in user frustration and a subsequent decline in engagement.

Concerns regarding privacy and security present considerable obstacles. Wearable devices produce extensive quantities of sensitive health data, rendering them appealing targets for cyberattacks. It is essential to guarantee robust data encryption, anonymization, and adherence to regulations such as the General Data

Protection Regulation (GDPR) and the Health Insurance Portability and Accountability Act (HIPAA) in order to sustain user trust and avert misuse.

Cost represents another significant factor that restricts access to wearable devices, particularly in low-resource settings. Although certain devices are affordable and readily accessible, others, such as continuous glucose monitors (CGMs) or sophisticated biosensors, continue to be prohibitively expensive for numerous patients. Addressing this disparity will require the implementation of targeted subsidies, the development of public-private partnerships, and the introduction of innovative business models that prioritize affordability and accessibility.

Ultimately, the challenges of integration can hinder the full potential of wearable devices in clinical care. Numerous devices operate independently, lacking interoperability with electronic health records (EHRs) or other healthcare platforms. Standardized protocols, such as those discussed in Chap. 2 (e.g., HL7 FHIR), are essential for establishing seamless ecosystems in which wearable data can enhance comprehensive patient care.

The Role of Wearables in Digital Medicine

Wearables and biosensors are not standalone innovations but integral components of the broader Digital Medicine ecosystem. Their ability to generate real-time, actionable data complements other digital tools, such as mHealth apps and artificial intelligence (AI) platforms. For example, a wearable device that tracks heart rate variability can feed data into an AI algorithm, which analyzes trends and predicts potential risks. This can prompt a mHealth app to suggest lifestyle adjustments or initiate a telemedicine consultation.

These technologies also exemplify the transition toward *P4 medicine*—predictive, preventive, personalized, and participatory. By empowering individuals to take responsibility for their health and providing clinicians with enhanced insights, wearable devices and biosensors contribute to a healthcare model that prioritizes long-term well-being over episodic interventions.

Looking Ahead

As wearable technology advances, its potential to transform healthcare grows exponentially. Miniaturization, improved sensor accuracy, and advancements in connectivity are paving the way for more comfortable, reliable, and accessible devices. Integrating wearables with AI and machine learning algorithms promises even more significant innovations, including predictive analytics that anticipate health issues before they arise.

Nevertheless, the realization of this vision necessitates collaborative efforts among stakeholders, which include technology developers, healthcare providers, policymakers, and patients. By addressing the challenges of affordability, interoperability, and privacy, we can ensure that wearables and biosensors fulfill their potential to enhance patient care and transform healthcare delivery.

Artificial Intelligence in Clinical Practice

Artificial intelligence (AI) has emerged as one of the most transformative forces in Digital Medicine, reshaping how clinicians interpret data, make decisions, and deliver care. Its capability to process vast and complex datasets, while uncovering patterns that may elude even the most proficient human observers, positions AI as an indispensable ally in contemporary healthcare. From diagnostics and predictive analytics to operational efficiency, AI propels the evolution of a healthcare model that is more precise, personalized, and proactive. This closely aligns with the foundational principles of Digital Medicine discussed in Chap. 2, which include the significance of data-driven care, clinical validation, and patient-centeredness.

Unlike many digital tools, artificial intelligence (AI) represents not merely a singular application but a multifaceted spectrum of technologies. These technologies range from rule-based algorithms to sophisticated machine learning (ML) systems that possess adaptive learning capabilities, thereby equipping AI to dynamically confront complex challenges within the healthcare sector. The applications of AI are deeply anchored in the fundamental principles of interoperability and data standards as elucidated in Chap. 2, which emphasize the significance of seamless data exchange and standardized frameworks for clinical tools.

Transformative Applications of AI in Medicine

Diagnostics: Enhancing Accuracy and Speed

As delineated in Chap. 2, Software as a Medical Device (SaMD) has redefined the conventional understanding of medical instruments by converting software into independent diagnostic systems. Artificial Intelligence further amplifies this transformation, facilitating unprecedented accuracy in the real-time analysis of clinical data. For instance, machine learning algorithms that have been trained on a multitude of imaging datasets possess the capability to detect subtle abnormalities in medical scans, such as early stage cancers or fractures, which human radiologists may inadvertently overlook.

A salient example previously examined is the integration of AI-powered imaging software within Digital Medicine platforms. These tools significantly enhance diagnostic accuracy and democratize access to expertise by rendering advanced diagnostic capabilities available to remote or underserved regions. This phenomenon exemplifies the overarching principle of accessibility, which was emphasized as a critical objective in Chap. 2.

Predictive Analytics: Proactive Healthcare

The transition from reactive to proactive care, as highlighted in the discussion of remote patient monitoring (RPM) in Chap. 2, finds its strongest ally in predictive analytics. Artificial intelligence (AI) has the capability to anticipate patient risks and facilitate early interventions by analyzing clinical data streams, outputs from wearable devices, and social determinants of health. For example, AI-driven models can forecast the onset of sepsis in hospitalized patients by examining subtle trends in vital signs. This capability aligns with the preventive and participatory aspects of P4 medicine.

Clinical Decision Support Systems (cDSS): Augmenting Human Expertise

In Chap. 2, interoperability and data standards have been recognized as essential enablers of tools that integrate effortlessly into clinical workflows. AI-powered clinical decision support systems (cDSS) exemplify this integration by synthesizing a variety of data sources to deliver evidence-based recommendations. For instance, oncology platforms that utilize AI to analyze tumor genomics, clinical guidelines, and real-world data empower clinicians to customize treatment plans to suit individual patients, thereby embodying the personalized aspect of P4 medicine.

Operational Efficiency: Optimizing Healthcare Systems

In addition to clinical care, artificial intelligence (AI) enhances operational efficiency by automating administrative tasks and optimizing resource allocation. Chapter 2 emphasized the role of digital tools in improving workflows, and AI builds upon this foundation by streamlining processes such as scheduling, patient inquiries, and resource forecasting. For instance, AI algorithms possess the capability to predict peak demand in emergency departments, thereby enabling hospitals to allocate staff and resources more effectively.

Digital Twins: Personalized Simulations

Chapter 2 introduces the concept of Digital Twins, which are virtual patient replicas and represent one of the most innovative applications of artificial intelligence (AI). By integrating data from electronic health records (EHRs), wearable devices, and biosensors, Digital Twins simulate disease progression, evaluate treatment options, and predict outcomes. This approach aligns with the principles of data-driven and adaptive care, demonstrating how AI enhances precision in personalized medicine.

Opportunities and Challenges

The opportunities and challenges presented by AI cover several themes addressed in Chap. 2, especially the ethical and regulatory concerns related to digital tools.

Opportunities

AI offers numerous opportunities to enhance care delivery:

Efficiency: The automation of repetitive tasks significantly contributes to the mitigation of clinician burnout, a concern that has also been previously emphasized during discussions regarding remote monitoring systems and mobile health (mHealth) applications.

Personalization: Algorithms specifically designed for individual patients facilitate more precise interventions, thereby reinforcing the personalized care strategies previously emphasized.

Scalability: AI systems process data at speeds and scales unmatched by human effort, supporting population health initiatives that align with the interoperability frameworks outlined in Chap. 2.

Challenges

Several challenges persist that are closely linked to the regulatory and ethical issues outlined previously:

Algorithmic Bias: As already discussed, the ethical utilization of artificial intelligence requires the incorporation of diverse training datasets to avert the perpetuation of disparities. It is imperative that AI systems undergo comprehensive validation processes to ensure inclusivity and fairness.

Explainability: The concept of trustworthy artificial intelligence, as delineated in Chap. 2 within the ethical guidelines, is imperative in this context. It is essential for clinicians and patients to understand the methodologies employed by AI systems in generating recommendations, thereby underscoring the necessity for the progression of explainable AI (XAI).

Regulatory Oversight: Frameworks such as the FDA's Software Pre-Cert Program, referenced in Chap. 2, are established to guarantee that AI tools adhere to rigorous safety and efficacy standards. However, the dynamic nature of AI presents ongoing challenges for regulators.

AI in the Broader Context of Digital Medicine

The transformative role of artificial intelligence (AI) in healthcare closely aligns with the foundational principles of Digital Medicine elaborated upon in Chap. 2. Its capacity to synthesize data from various sources—such as electronic health records (EHRs), wearable devices, biosensors, and patient-reported outcomes—illustrates the interconnected nature of Digital Health tools. For example, an AI algorithm that analyzes real-time heart rate variability data from a wearable device can trigger an alert to a telemedicine platform, thereby initiating a virtual consultation. This integration exemplifies how AI enhances accessibility, efficiency, and personalization—key themes interwoven throughout this book.

Moreover, artificial intelligence contributes to the overarching goals of predictive and preventive healthcare by identifying potential risks prior to their progression into significant health concerns. These capabilities exemplify the synergy between artificial intelligence and other digital tools, including remote patient monitoring systems and biosensors, which supply the continuous data streams essential for effective AI-driven analytics.

Looking Ahead: The Future of AI in Medicine

The integration of AI into clinical practice represents not only a technological advancement but also a cultural transformation in how healthcare is delivered. As AI continues to evolve, its applications will encompass emerging trends such as generative AI for drug discovery, augmented reality (AR) for precision surgery, and AI-driven chatbots for mental health support. These innovations are congruent with the principles of adaptive and dynamic care, first introduced in Chap. 2.

Nonetheless, the realization of artificial intelligence's full potential necessitates continuous collaboration among diverse stakeholders, including clinicians, data scientists, policymakers, and patients. It is imperative to address issues of bias, transparency, and integration to ensure that AI not only enhances clinical practice but also safeguards patient trust and promotes equity. By upholding the foundational principles of Digital Medicine, we can leverage AI as a formidable instrument for the transformation of healthcare and the enhancement of patient outcomes.

Looking Ahead: Convergence of Technologies

As Digital Medicine continues to evolve, the convergence of various technologies—including telemedicine, mobile health (mHealth) applications, wearable devices, biosensors, and artificial intelligence (AI)—heralds the advent of a more integrated and patient-centered healthcare ecosystem. This convergence constitutes not only a technical advancement but also signifies a philosophical transition toward a proactive, personalized, and participatory model of care. Building upon the foundational concepts introduced in Chap. 2, such as interoperability, clinical validation, and patient empowerment, this section examines how the amalgamation of digital tools enhances healthcare delivery while addressing the complexities of integration.

Synergistic Models for Future Healthcare

The integration of digital tools into a cohesive system promises to dismantle the silos that have traditionally fragmented healthcare. Imagine a scenario where a wearable biosensor detects subtle changes in a patient's vital signs, triggering an AI-powered analytics platform to identify potential risks. This analysis, in turn, prompts a notification to both the patient and their healthcare provider through a mobile health (mHealth) app, leading to a virtual telemedicine consultation. Such seamless interoperability creates a unified care pathway, aligning with the principles of *data-driven decision-making* and *patient-cenetred design* outlined in Chap. 2.

For instance, in the management of chronic conditions such as diabetes, integrated platforms may combine continuous glucose monitoring (CGM) data sourced from wearable devices, behavioral insights derived from mobile health applications, and predictive algorithms enabled by artificial intelligence (AI). This system is poised to provide real-time recommendations meticulously tailored to the individual's lifestyle and health objectives, thereby embodying the personalized and participatory dimensions of P4 medicine as introduced in Chap. 1. Similarly, in acute care environments, such integration has the potential to enable quicker and more accurate triage, consequently reducing delays in diagnosis and treatment.

This convergence extends beyond clinical care; it also encompasses public health initiatives, wherein aggregated data from wearable devices and Digital Health applications can yield insights at the population level. For example, artificial intelligence algorithms have the capability to analyze trends in symptom reports submitted through mobile health platforms during a public health crisis to forecast outbreak patterns, thereby facilitating targeted interventions. These applications emphasize the potential for scalable and adaptive healthcare systems, a recurring theme throughout this guide.

The Role of Interoperability in Convergence

As emphasized in Chap. 2, *interoperability and data standards* constitute the foundation of Digital Medicine. It is imperative that data flows seamlessly across platforms, devices, and healthcare systems to facilitate the successful convergence of technologies. Standards such as HL7 FHIR (Fast Healthcare Interoperability Resources) and SNOMED CT provide the common language and infrastructure essential for the integration of diverse tools into a cohesive ecosystem.

In the absence of interoperability, the complete potential of convergence remains unfulfilled. Fragmented systems lead to unnecessary data collection, inconsistencies in patient records, and delays in clinical decision-making. By prioritizing open standards and fostering cross-sector collaboration, healthcare stakeholders have the capacity to address these challenges and create a truly connected digital ecosystem.

Challenges and Opportunities

Although the convergence of technologies presents considerable promise, it also introduces distinct challenges that must be addressed to ensure equitable and sustainable adoption.

Data Privacy and Security

The integration of diverse technologies enhances the volume and sensitivity of patient data collected, stored, and shared, consequently elevating substantial concerns regarding privacy and cybersecurity. As elaborated in Chap. 2, frameworks such as *the General Data Protection R*egulation (GDPR) and the *Health Insurance*

*Portability and Accoun*tability Act (HIPAA) delineate guidelines for the protection of patient information; nevertheless, the ever-evolving characteristics of digital ecosystems demand ongoing vigilance and innovation in data governance.

Equity and Accessibility

The digital divide continues to pose a significant challenge. Populations in low-resource settings or with limited digital literacy frequently encounter difficulties in accessing or leveraging advanced digital tools. It is imperative to ensure that convergent technologies are both affordable and user-friendly in order to avert disparities in healthcare outcomes. Initiatives such as government subsidies, public-private partnerships, and community education programs can play a pivotal role in bridging these gaps.

Cost and Sustainability

The integration of technologies necessitates a substantial investment in infrastructure, training, and maintenance. Healthcare organizations must conduct a thorough assessment of the long-term sustainability of convergent systems, balancing initial costs with potential benefits, such as improved outcomes, operational efficiency, and cost savings.

Ethical Considerations

As multiple technologies converge, ethical dilemmas become increasingly complex. For instance, who possesses the data generated by integrated platforms? How can we guarantee that AI algorithms prioritise patient welfare over commercial interests? Tackling these questions necessitates robust ethical guidelines, such as those discussed in Chap. 2.3 on privacy and bias.

A Vision for the Future

The convergence of telemedicine, mHealth apps, wearables, and AI signifies more than just a technological evolution; it marks a paradigm shift in how healthcare is delivered and experienced. By integrating these tools into a cohesive system, healthcare providers can transition from reactive care to a predictive, preventive, and personalized model.

This future envisions a healthcare ecosystem where technologies collaborate and adapt flexibly to the needs of individual patients and populations. For instance, an AI-powered platform may analyze trends across wearable data, mHealth app usage, and telemedicine consultations to pinpoint gaps in care delivery. Such insights could inform targeted interventions, ensuring timely and effective care.

Furthermore, incorporating these tools into population health strategies could facilitate a transition toward *precision public health*, where interventions are customized for specific communities or demographics. By utilizing aggregated data from Digital Health platforms, policymakers could distribute resources more efficiently, tackling health disparities and enhancing societal outcomes.

Convergence as a Pillar of Digital Medicine

As explored in Chap. 1, Digital Medicine is not merely a collection of isolated innovations but rather an evolving ecosystem that demands collaboration, adaptability, and innovation. The convergence of technologies exemplifies this vision, creating a healthcare model that prioritizes patient engagement, clinical precision, and system-wide efficiency. However, achieving this vision requires a collective commitment to overcoming technical, ethical, and logistical challenges.

By promoting collaboration among technologists, clinicians, policymakers, and patients, we can ensure that the convergence of digital tools realizes its promise of transforming healthcare into a more connected, equitable, and patient-centered enterprise. As the field of Digital Medicine continues to advance, this integration will serve as a cornerstone for its future, bridging the gap between technological potential and real-world impact.

Case Studies and Practical Exercises

Case Studies

Case Study #1: Kaiser Permanente's Telehealth Model

Summary: Kaiser Permanente incorporates telemedicine into primary care workflows, resulting in a 40% decrease in in-person visits while upholding high levels of patient satisfaction.

Key Takeaways: Efficiency, cost reduction, and importance of reimbursement policies.

Case Study #2: MySugr—Diabetes Management App

Summary: MySugr uses gamification, AI-driven coaching, and real-time glucose tracking to improve diabetes self-management.

Key Takeaways: Patient engagement, data integration, AI-driven decision support.

Case Study #3: Apple Watch & AFib Detection

Summary: The ECG feature of the Apple Watch allows for early detection of atrial fibrillation, encouraging users to consult medical care prior to experiencing symptoms worsening.

Key Takeaways: Real-world impact of wearables, regulatory classification, public adoption challenges.

Case Study #4: IBM Watson for Oncology

Summary: IBM Watson applies AI-driven decision support to oncology, offering treatment recommendations based on real-world patient data.
Key Takeaways: AI bias, clinician trust, scalability.

Practical Exercises

Exercise #1: Designing a Telemedicine Workflow Select a patient population (e.g., rural elderly, post-operative patients). Outline a telehealth workflow, taking into accounttriage, consultation, and follow-up.

Reflection Question: How would you ensure equitable access to telehealth services?

Exercise #2: Evaluating an mHealth App Choose an mHealth app (e.g., a mental health chatbot, medication tracker). Evaluate usability, effectiveness, and regulatory compliance.

Reflection Question: How can mHealth apps reconcile accessibility with clinical rigor?

Exercise #3: Wearable Data Integration in Clinical Practice Envisage a scenario where wearable data (e.g., blood pressure monitor) must be integrated into an HER, possibly using AI instances. Define the technical and clinical requirements for data interoperability.

Reflection Question: What steps can be taken to ensure fairness in AI-driven healthcare?

Final Thoughts

By incorporating these real-world case studies, exercises, and reflection questions, we enhance the book's practical value while maintaining its academic rigor. These elements promote active learning, making it a more engaging and applicable resource for clinicians, administrators, and policymakers navigating Digital Medicine.

Suggested Reading

1. U.S. Food and Drug Administration (FDA). Telemedicine policies and practices for remote care. FDA Digital Health Center of Excellence. 2023. Retrieved from https://www.fda.gov.
2. World Health Organization (WHO). mHealth: new horizons for health through mobile technologies. In: Global observatory for eHealth Series, vol. 3; 2022. Retrieved from https://www.who.int.

3. Digital Therapeutics Alliance (DTA). Advancing the adoption of digital health technologies. Digital Therapeutics Alliance Resources. 2023. Retrieved from https://dtxalliance.org.
4. Topol EJ. Deep medicine: how artificial intelligence can make healthcare human again. New York: Basic Books; 2019.
5. HealthIT.gov. Interoperability and the integration of wearables and mHealth tools into EHRs. HealthIT Articles. 2023. Retrieved from https://www.healthit.gov.
6. European Commission. Ethical guidelines for artificial intelligence in digital medicine. 2022. Retrieved from https://ec.europa.eu.
7. McKinsey & Company. Convergence in digital health: harnessing the power of integration. Healthcare Insights; 2023. Retrieved from https://www.mckinsey.com.
8. MIT Technology Review. The role of AI in preventive healthcare. MIT Technology Review Articles. 2023. Retrieved from https://www.technologyreview.com.
9. National Health Service (NHS). Integrating mHealth into public health programs. NHS Digital Innovations Report. 2023. Retrieved from https://www.nhs.uk.
10. Cesario A, et al. Personalized medicine meets artificial intelligence: beyond the hype towards the Metaverse. Springer; 2023.
11. World Health Organization. mHealth: new horizons for health through mobile technologies, Global Observatory for eHealth Series, vol. 3; 2011. Retrieved from http://apps.who.int/iris/bitstream/handle/10665/44607/9789241564250_eng.pdf?sequence=1.
12. World Health Organization. WHO guideline: recommendations on digital interventions for health system strengthening. 2019. Retrieved from https://www.who.int/publications/i/item/9789241550505.
13. World Health Organization. Global strategy on digital health 2020–2025. 2021. Retrieved from https://www.who.int/publications/i/item/9789240020924.
14. World Health Organization. Ethics and governance of artificial intelligence for health. 2021. Retrieved from https://www.who.int/publications/i/item/9789240029200.
15. European Commission. Enabling the digital transformation of health and care in the Digital Single Market; empowering citizens and building a healthier society. (COM (2018) 233 final). 2018. Retrieved from https://eur-lex.europa.eu/legal-content/EN/TXT/?uri=COM:2018:233:FIN.
16. Topol, E. Preparing the healthcare workforce to deliver the digital future. (The Topol Review) Health Education England. 2019. Retrieved from https://topol.hee.nhs.uk/wp-content/uploads/HEE-Topol-Review-2019.pdf.
17. Office of the National Coordinator for Health Information Technology (ONC). 21st Century Cures Act: interoperability, information blocking, and the ONC Health IT Certification Program (Final Rule). 2020. Retrieved from https://www.healthit.gov/sites/default/files/cures/2020-03/ONC_Cures_Act_Final_Rule_03092020.pdf.
18. Health Level Seven International (HL7). 2019. HL7 publishes FHIR® Release 4. Retrieved from https://blog.hl7.org/hl7-publishes-fhir-release-4.
19. Koonin LM, Hoots B, Tsang CA, et al. Trends in the use of telehealth during the emergence of the COVID-19 pandemic — United States, January–March 2020. MMWR Morb Mortal Wkly Rep. 2020;69(43):1595–9. Retrieved from https://www.cdc.gov/mmwr/volumes/69/wr/mm6943a3.htm.
20. Kuan PX, Chan WK, Ying DKF, et al. Efficacy of telemedicine for the management of cardiovascular disease: a systematic review and meta-analysis. Lancet Digit Health. 2022;4(9):e676–91. Retrieved from https://pubmed.ncbi.nlm.nih.gov/36028290/.
21. World Health Organization. (2010). Telemedicine: opportunities and developments in member states (Global observatory for eHealth series, Vol. 2). Retrieved from https://apps.who.int/iris/handle/10665/44497.
22. Patel NA, Butte AJ. Characteristics and challenges of the clinical pipeline of digital therapeutics. NPJ Digit Med. 2020;3:159. Retrieved from https://www.nature.com/articles/s41746-020-00370-8

23. Dang A, Arora D, Rane P. Role of digital therapeutics and the changing future of healthcare. J Family Med Prim Care. 2020;9(5):2207–13. Retrieved from https://www.ncbi.nlm.nih.gov/pmc/articles/PMC7444649/.
24. Food and Drug Administration (FDA). Artificial Intelligence/Machine Learning (AI/ML)-based software as a medical device action plan. 2021. Retrieved from https://www.fda.gov/media/145022/download.
25. Topol EJ. High-performance medicine: the convergence of human and artificial intelligence. Nat Med. 2019;25(1):44–56. Retrieved from https://pubmed.ncbi.nlm.nih.gov/30617339/.
26. Jiang F, Jiang Y, Zhi H, et al. Artificial intelligence in healthcare: past, present and future. Stroke Vasc Neurol. 2017;2(4):230–43. Retrieved from https://svn.bmj.com/content/2/4/230.
27. Richardson S, Lawrence K, Schoenthaler AM, et al. A framework for digital health equity. NPJ Digit Med. 2022;5:119. Retrieved from https://www.nature.com/articles/s41746-022-00663-0.
28. Babu M, Lautman Z, Lin X, et al. Wearable devices: implications for precision medicine and the future of health care. Annu Rev Med. 2024;75:401–15. Retrieved from https://doi.org/10.1146/annurev-med-052422-020437.
29. Lu L, Zhang J, Xie Y, et al. Wearable health devices in health care: narrative systematic review. JMIR Mhealth Uhealth. 2020;8(11):e18907. Retrieved from https://mhealth.jmir.org/2020/11/e18907/.
30. Wang G, Badal A, Jia X, et al. Development of metaverse for intelligent healthcare. Nat Mach Intell. 2022;4:922–9. Retrieved from https://doi.org/10.1038/s42256-022-00549-6.
31. Kickbusch I, Piselli D, Agrawal A, et al. The Lancet and Financial Times Commission on governing health futures 2030: growing up in a digital world. Lancet. 2021;398(10312):1727–76. Retrieved from https://pubmed.ncbi.nlm.nih.gov/34678103/.
32. Dorsey ER, Topol EJ. Telemedicine 2020 and the next decade. Lancet. 2020;395(10227):859. Retrieved from https://pubmed.ncbi.nlm.nih.gov/32171399/.
33. Budd J, Miller BS, Manning EM, et al. Digital technologies in the public-health response to COVID-19. Nat Med. 2020;26(8):1183–92. Retrieved from https://pubmed.ncbi.nlm.nih.gov/32770165/.
34. National Health Service (NHS). The NHS long term plan. 2019. Retrieved from https://www.longtermplan.nhs.uk/wp-content/uploads/2019/08/nhs-long-term-plan-version-1.2.pdf.
35. Rivas H, Wac K, editors. Digital health: scaling healthcare to the world. Cham: Springer; 2018.
36. Marcolino MS, Oliveira JAQ, D'Agostino M, et al. The impact of mHealth interventions: systematic review of systematic reviews. JMIR Mhealth Uhealth. 2018;6(1):e23. Retrieved from https://mhealth.jmir.org/2018/1/e23/.
37. Liu X, Faes L, Kale AU, et al. A comparison of deep learning performance against healthcare professionals in detecting diseases from medical imaging: a systematic review and meta-analysis. Lancet Digit Health. 2019;1(6):e271–97. Retrieved from https://pubmed.ncbi.nlm.nih.gov/33323251/.
38. Meskó B, Győrffy Z. The rise of the empowered physician in the digital health era. J Med Internet Res. 2019;21(3):e12490. Retrieved from https://www.jmir.org/2019/3/e12490/.
39. Organisation for Economic Co-operation and Development (OECD). Health in the 21st century: putting data to work for stronger health systems. Paris: OECD Publishing; 2019. Retrieved from https://doi.org/10.1787/e3b23f8e-en.
40. Greenhalgh T, Wherton J, Papoutsi C, et al. Beyond adoption: a new framework for theorizing and evaluating nonadoption, abandonment, and challenges to the scale-up of health and care technologies. J Med Internet Res. 2017;19(11):e367. Retrieved from https://www.jmir.org/2017/11/e367/.
41. World Health Organization & International Telecommunication Union. National eHealth strategy toolkit. Geneva: WHO Press; 2012. Retrieved from https://apps.who.int/iris/handle/10665/75211.
42. Matheny ME, Israni ST, Ahmed MN, Whicher D, editors. Artificial intelligence in health care: the hope, the hype, the promise, the peril. Washington: National Academy of Medicine; 2019. Retrieved from https://nam.edu/wp-content/uploads/2019/12/AI-in-Health-Care-PREPUB-FINAL.pdf.

43. Vayena E, Haeusermann T, Adjekum A, Blasimme A. Digital health: meeting the ethical and policy challenges. Swiss Med Wkly. 2018;148:w14571. Retrieved from https://pubmed.ncbi.nlm.nih.gov/29376547/.
44. Department of Health and Social Care (UK). A guide to good practice for digital and data-driven health technologies. 2021. Retrieved from https://www.gov.uk/government/publications/code-of-conduct-for-data-driven-health-and-care-technology/initial-code-of-conduct-for-data-driven-health-and-care-technology.

Implementing Digital Medicine in Clinical Practice

4

Assessing Organizational Needs and Goals

The foundation of any successful Digital Medicine initiative is a clear understanding of the organization's needs and goals. Implementing digital tools is not merely a technological upgrade but a targeted effort to address real-world issues, enhance care delivery, and align with broader institutional priorities. Evaluating these needs necessitates a candid assessment of clinical challenges, operational inefficiencies, and opportunities to improve patient engagement.

The first step is to identify and define the core challenges that digital solutions aim to address. These challenges can vary widely depending on the organization's specific context but generally fall into three main categories: clinical priorities, operational inefficiencies, and gaps in patient engagement.

Identifying Core Challenges

Identifying core challenges is the initial step in aligning digital tools with significant outcomes. Without this clarity, organizations risk adopting technology for its own sake instead of addressing pressing issues.

For many organizations, clinical priorities are the main drivers of digital adoption. For example, a hospital managing a high volume of chronic heart failure patients might deploy remote patient monitoring (RPM) devices to provide real-time insights into patient health. These tools can alert clinicians to early signs of decompensation, preventing costly hospital readmissions and improving patient outcomes. Similarly, a clinic addressing high rates of uncontrolled diabetes might implement digital therapeutics to provide patients with personalized guidance on diet, exercise, and medication adherence.

Operational inefficiencies are a common pain point. High no-show rates, administrative bottlenecks, and resource constraints can weigh heavily on healthcare

A. Cesario et al., *Digital Medicine Starter Guide*,
https://doi.org/10.1007/978-3-032-01272-2_4

systems. For instance, telemedicine platforms enable patients to attend consultations from their homes, minimizing missed appointments and optimizing provider schedules.

Engaging patients more effectively is also a cornerstone of Digital Medicine. Wearable devices and mHealth applications empower patients to take a more active role in managing their health, thereby fostering better adherence to care plans. For instance, wearable ECG devices can assist patients in monitoring their cardiac health while providing clinicians with continuous data to guide treatment.

Examining these challenges and their root causes can help organizations develop targeted digital strategies. For example, a rural clinic might prioritize telemedicine to address transportation barriers, while an urban academic hospital could focus on AI-driven diagnostic tools to streamline radiology workflows.

Readiness Checks and Resource Inventory

After identifying challenges, organizations must evaluate their readiness to implement digital solutions. This entails assessing infrastructure, workforce capabilities, and financial resources to ensure a robust foundation for success.

Infrastructure Readiness

Technological infrastructure acts as the backbone of Digital Medicine. Organizations must ensure that networks are dependable, devices are compatible, and systems are interoperable. For instance, hospitals adopting wearable ECG patches must confirm that these devices integrate seamlessly with their electronic health record (EHR) systems, enabling clinicians to access and interpret the data within existing workflows. Standards such as HL7 FHIR, discussed in Chap. 2, are essential for facilitating this interoperability.

Furthermore, network reliability is crucial for telemedicine platforms. Patients in remote areas with limited internet connectivity may struggle to access virtual consultations, undermining the platform's effectiveness. Promptly addressing these gaps can prevent implementation setbacks.

Workforce Competencies

Digital tools are only as effective as the individuals who utilize them. Organizations must assess the digital literacy of their workforce and provide training to rectify any deficiencies. For instance, nurses managing RPM programs may need to learn how to interpret data trends, set alert thresholds, and respond effectively to deviations. Similarly, radiologists using AI tools for diagnostics should be trained to validate algorithm outputs and recognize potential biases.

Extended Example: A regional hospital that implemented an AI-powered triage tool for its emergency departments found that staff were unfamiliar with interpreting AI risk scores. The hospital collaborated with technology vendors to organize workshops, equipping clinicians with the knowledge necessary to confidently integrate AI insights into their decision-making processes.

Financial Sustainability

The digital transformation of healthcare necessitates substantial financial investments that transcend the initial acquisition of technologies. Organizations are required to allocate resources for workforce training, system integration, cybersecurity measures, ongoing maintenance, and future scalability. These aggregated costs can impose a considerable burden on healthcare systems, especially those operating under stringent public budgets or within fragmented governance frameworks.

In this context, funding models assume critical importance. Exploring diversified financial pathways—such as national and European grants, performance-based investment schemes, and strategic public-private partnerships—can contribute to mitigating financial strain and facilitating the acceleration of innovation uptake. These instruments are particularly pertinent in countries with universal health coverage models, where financial stewardship must strike a balance between innovation and equity.

The Italian National Health Service (SSN) exemplifies a paradigmatic case. As a universalist and tax-funded system grounded in the principles of equity, solidarity, and subsidiarity, the SSN offers a distinctive governance structure wherein regional authorities are entrusted with the implementation of nationally defined essential levels of care (LEA—Livelli Essenziali di Assistenza). This decentralized framework presents both challenges and opportunities for the sustainable adoption of digital medicine. On the one hand, regional heterogeneity may hinder uniform deployment; conversely, it enables context-sensitive experimentation and grassroots innovation. Financial sustainability, in this context, relies not only on national allocation mechanisms but also on the regions' capacity to integrate digital health into existing care pathways and performance metrics.

More broadly, health systems anchored in universalism and subsidiarity, such as those prevalent across much of continental Europe, must ensure that digital investments are aligned with long-term goals of accessibility, inclusion, and social justice. In these models, cost-effectiveness and value-based procurement serve as essential levers to guarantee that digital tools do not exacerbate existing inequities but, rather, contribute to bridging gaps in care delivery and enhancing system responsiveness.

As elaborated in Chap. 3, the increasing availability of reimbursement frameworks for telemedicine and remote patient monitoring (RPM)—comprising national codes and tariff structures—significantly supports the financial viability of digital interventions. In Italy, although reimbursement for telehealth services is progressing, the full integration into standard care models remains inconsistent across regions, revealing an ongoing need for policy harmonization and fiscal incentives that prioritize scalable, evidence-based solutions.

Extended Example: A large outpatient center piloting a digital therapeutic platform for diabetes management secured funding through a government grant and a partnership with a technology provider. The program demonstrated a significant reduction in HbA1c levels among participants, resulting in additional funding for expansion.

Addressing these areas of readiness—technology, workforce, and finances—can aid organizations in facilitating smoother implementation and achieving a more substantial impact.

Selecting the Right Digital Tools

The next crucial step in implementing Digital Medicine involves identifying the appropriate tools. After evaluating organizational needs and readiness, the focus shifts to selecting solutions that are in line with clinical goals, operational workflows, and patient engagement priorities.

Aligning Technology with Clinical Goals

The process of selecting digital tools begins with identifying how they will address the specific challenges outlined in the needs assessment. Digital tools should resolve issues and align with broader organizational strategies. For example:

- A hospital seeking to reduce readmissions for chronic heart failure might concentrate on RPM tools that provide real-time alerts and integrate with EHR systems.
- A primary care clinic encountering challenges with medication adherence might opt for mHealth applications that offer automated reminders and personalized interventions for patients.

Key considerations include:

Clinical Validation: Tools must demonstrate their effectiveness through peer-reviewed studies and regulatory approvals.

User-Friendly Design: Platforms should feature intuitive interfaces that minimize learning curves for both clinicians and patients.

Scalability: Solutions must accommodate future growth, whether in patient volume or data complexity.

Customizing Solutions vs. Off-the-Shelf Products

Organizations must determine whether to adopt off-the-shelf tools or invest in bespoke solutions tailored to their specific workflows.

Off-the-Shelf Tools

Ready-made solutions facilitate rapid implementation and vendor support. For example, telemedicine platforms with pre-built video consultation features can effectively address high no-show rates. These tools are often verified, reliable, and cost-effective.

Customized Solutions

Tailored solutions offer flexibility and alignment with specific organizational requirements. For example, a hospital system adopting AI imaging tools might opt for a custom platform to guarantee smooth integration with its radiology infrastructure, providing comprehensive control over data security and workflow design.

By carefully evaluating these options, organizations can select tools that balance ease of implementation with long-term flexibility.

Integration with EHR and Data Workflow

The seamless integration of digital tools with electronic health record (EHR) systems constitutes a fundamental aspect of Digital Medicine. EHRs serve as the central repository for patient information, and it is imperative that new technologies interface seamlessly with these systems to augment care delivery and avert data silos. Such effective integration optimizes clinical workflows and equips healthcare providers with comprehensive, real-time insights.

Workflow Adjustments

Adopting new digital tools generally necessitates significant modifications to established workflows. While the promise of enhanced efficiency and better patient care is appealing, integrating new data streams demands meticulous planning and a realignment of roles within clinical teams.

Redefining Roles

The influx of data from wearable devices, telehealth platforms, or AI-driven tools creates the need for clear responsibilities in data management. For example, a hospital implementing wearable ECG patches must determine who will review and triage the incoming data. In some instances, this may involve creating new roles, such as digital navigators, responsible for managing data streams and escalating actionable insights to clinicians. This ensures that providers are not overwhelmed by information while maintaining a proactive approach to patient care.

Alert Management

Automated alerts represent a significant feature of numerous digital tools; however, they can become a double-edged sword if not calibrated appropriately. Excessively sensitive thresholds may lead to false positives, thereby inducing “alert fatigue” among staff, who may subsequently overlook critical notifications. Customizing alerts to prioritize clinically significant data—such as sustained abnormal heart rates identified by wearable devices—facilitates the achievement of a balance between sensitivity and relevance, ensuring that clinicians concentrate on actionable issues.

Streamlining Documentation

The integration of new data streams into electronic health record (EHR) systems is anticipated to enhance documentation workflows rather than impede them. For instance, summaries from telehealth visits should automatically populate structured fields within the EHR, thereby conserving time and ensuring consistency. It is imperative for organizations to collaborate closely with vendors to design interfaces that facilitate seamless data entry while minimizing disruptions to clinical routines.

Adjustments to workflows should be approached iteratively, incorporating regular feedback from staff to address challenges and optimize processes. The ensuing sections will elucidate the significance of training and engagement, which are equally essential for promoting adoption and ensuring sustainability.

Addressing Common Implementation Hurdles

Digital transformation seldom progresses without hurdles. Common challenges include maintaining data security, tackling staff resistance, and managing change fatigue; however, appropriate strategies can overcome these.

Security and Privacy Concerns

As Digital Medicine expands the types and volume of data collected, safeguarding patient information becomes ever more critical. Trust is the foundation of successful digital adoption, and even a single data breach can threaten relationships with patients and stakeholders.

Ensuring Compliance

Adhering to regulatory frameworks such as the GDPR, HIPAA, and MDR is essential. Compliance audits should be conducted regularly to ensure that digital tools meet security standards. For instance, AI platforms that process imaging data must implement robust safeguards to prevent unauthorized access or inadvertent data leaks.

Building Secure Systems

End-to-end encryption guarantees that sensitive information remains secure during both transmission and storage. Role-based access controls limit data visibility to authorized personnel, thereby minimizing the risk of internal breaches. For instance, a telemedicine platform might provide physicians, administrative staff, and IT teams with varying levels of access depending on their specific roles.

Incident Response Planning

Organizations must also be prepared to respond quickly to potential breaches. A clear incident response plan—covering containment, notification, and root cause analysis—can minimize damage and showcase accountability. Transparency in managing such events helps maintain trust and reassures patients of the organization's dedication to privacy.

Staff Engagement and Change Fatigue

Resistance to new technologies often stems from fear of the unknown or concerns about increased workloads. To tackle this, organizations must prioritize transparency, training, and collaboration.

Transparent Communication

Staff must understand the reasons behind digital initiatives. Clear communication regarding the benefits of new tools—such as decreased diagnostic workloads or enhanced patient engagement—can help alleviate scepticism and cultivate enthusiasm.

Building Internal Champions

Digital champions—respected colleagues advocating for new technology—play a crucial role in encouraging acceptance. By mentoring their peers and showcasing the tools' value in practical scenarios, these champions can expedite adoption and reduce resistance.

Phased Implementation

Incremental rollouts allow organizations to refine workflows and address challenges before scaling up. For example, a hospital might pilot an AI-based triage tool in one department, using the insights gained to improve training and protocols prior to broader deployment.

Change Management and Continuous Training

Sustained success in Digital Medicine necessitates a cultural shift that embraces innovation, continuous learning, and collaboration at all organizational levels.

Fostering a Digital Culture

Leadership is crucial for cultivating a culture of innovation. Leaders can instil confidence and commitment within the team by consistently aligning digital initiatives with patient-centered objectives. Regular meetings to celebrate achievements, address challenges, and realign on common goals reinforce the organization's vision.

Creating Incentives for Growth

Providing formal certifications, professional development opportunities, or recognition programs encourages staff to enhance their digital skills. For instance, clinicians may pursue certifications in AI ethics or telehealth best practices that are backed by organizational resources.

Tailoring Training Programs

Training should be accessible, practical, and tailored to meet the diverse needs of staff.

Hands-On Learning

Workshops and simulations provide clinicians with practical experience, such as interpreting AI-generated insights or conducting virtual consultations. These sessions enhance their confidence and competence in utilizing new tools.

On-Demand Resources

Flexible learning options, such as e-learning modules and recorded webinars, guarantee that all staff can access training regardless of their schedules.

Peer Mentorship

Pairing experienced users with newcomers fosters a supportive learning environment and promotes skill development throughout the team.

Measuring Impact and Sustainability

The long-term success of Digital Medicine relies on assessing its impact and adapting to changing needs. Key metrics provide insights into whether initiatives are achieving their intended goals and highlight opportunities for improvement.

Defining Key Performance Indicators (KPIs)

When evaluating the impact of digital health, traditional metrics often fall short. The transformation underway is not just technological but systemic, demanding a more nuanced set of indicators—ones capable of capturing clinical value, operational efficiency, long-term sustainability, and social legitimacy.

In this context, key performance indicators (KPIs) serve as strategic instruments. They help organizations determine whether digital interventions are truly improving care, making systems more responsive, and enhancing experiences for both patients and professionals. But KPIs must also help answer broader questions: are these innovations sustainable, equitable, and trustworthy?

Clinical Health Impact Metrics

Digital tools should not merely digitalize existing routines; rather, they should lead to tangible improvements in health outcomes. Clinical key performance indicators (KPIs) may include reductions in hospital readmissions for chronic conditions such as heart failure or chronic obstructive pulmonary disease (COPD), enhancements in disease-specific markers, exemplified by HbA1c levels in diabetic patients, or the earlier detection of complications facilitated by remote monitoring.

Additional relevant indicators underscore the expanded access to care enabled by telemedicine platforms or mobile health applications, as well as increased adherence to treatment regimens bolstered by digital engagement. Patient safety constitutes another critical dimension, often evaluated through the reduction of clinical errors attributable to decision-support systems and improved continuity of care.

Economic Sustainability Metrics

Digital transformation necessitates significant investment—not solely in hardware and software but also in training, workflows, and organizational change. Economic key performance indicators (KPIs) are fundamental for evaluating whether these investments yield value. These may encompass reductions in overall system costs, enhancements in the cost-effectiveness of specific digital solutions, or improvements in productivity and workflow efficiency, such as decreased wait times or optimized diagnostics.

In national health systems such as Italy's Servizio Sanitario Nazionale (SSN), where services are universally provided and organized through regional authorities, financial sustainability must also consider the capacity to scale digital health equitably. This encompasses strategic investments in digital infrastructure and capacity-building across diverse local contexts.

Technical Sustainability Metrics

Sustainable digital health depends on robust, secure, and future-ready technology. KPIs in this category assess system uptime, interoperability between platforms, and the scalability of solutions over time. Data protection and compliance—particularly with frameworks such as the General Data Protection Regulation (GDPR)—are fundamental benchmarks, as are metrics related to cybersecurity breaches and incident responses.

User accessibility also plays a central role: are platforms intuitive, compatible with Sustainable digital health fundamentally depends on robust, secure, and future-ready technology. Key performance indicators (KPIs) in this domain evaluate system uptime, interoperability between platforms, and the scalability of solutions over time. Data protection and compliance—particularly with regulatory frameworks such as the General Data Protection Regulation (GDPR)—are essential benchmarks, along with metrics pertaining to cybersecurity breaches and incident responses.

Accessibility for users also occupies a central role: Are platforms intuitive, compatible with widely used devices, and usable by individuals with varying levels of digital literacy? Technical sustainability is concerned with ensuring that tools are not only functional but also usable, adaptable, and resilient literacy? Technical sustainability is ultimately about ensuring that tools are not only functional but also usable, adaptable, and resilient.

Social Sustainability Metrics

This final set of Key performance indicators (KPIs) may be considered the most complex, yet simultaneously the most crucial. In health systems founded upon the principles of universalism and subsidiarity, such as the National Health Service (NHS), social sustainability is not merely ancillary; it constitutes a core objective. The metrics in this context examine whether digital tools are equitably accessible to all segments of the population, or whether there is a risk of exacerbating existing disparities.

Additionally, these metrics assess how patients and professionals perceive and experience digital health through various mechanisms, including satisfaction surveys, acceptance rates, and feedback loops. Further KPIs could monitor the degree of community engagement in the co-design of services, the impact of technology on workforce well-being—encompassing elements such as burnout and job satisfaction—and even broader cultural shifts in how individuals relate to healthcare, exemplified by the emergence of more participatory or preventive health behaviors.

Significantly, these metrics aid in capturing the less visible yet equally critical dimension of trust: how citizens perceive the management of their data, the transparency of digital processes, and the integrity of the institutions deploying these tools.

By incorporating KPIs across these four domains—clinical, economic, technical, and social—one can achieve a more comprehensive understanding of what success in digital health truly entails. This approach enables systems to transcend mere adoption and advance toward genuine transformation—one that is sustainable, inclusive, and aligned with the foundational values that underpin public health.

Case Studies and Practical Exercises

Case Studies

Case Study #1: Mayo Clinic's Digital Transformation Strategy

Summary: The Mayo Clinic has crafted a multi-year digital transformation roadmap designed to integrate AI, telemedicine, and remote monitoring into patient care. This strategy is founded on an internal needs assessment, an evaluation of the infrastructure, and a phased deployment approach intended to minimize disruption.

Key Takeaways: The importance of aligning technology with institutional priorities, conducting readiness assessments, and securing leadership buy-in.

Case Study #2: Cleveland Clinic's AI-Driven Radiology Implementation

Summary: The Cleveland Clinic has implemented AI-assisted radiology tools to enhance diagnostic accuracy and workflow efficiency. The hospital selected a commercial AI imaging solution that has been validated by peer-reviewed studies and integrated it with their existing PACS and EHR systems.

Key Takeaways: Importance of clinical validation, balancing customization vs. *off-the-shelf tools, ensuring seamless integration with existing workflows.*

Case Study #3: The Netherlands' Nationwide EHR Interoperability Initiative

Summary: The Dutch healthcare system has launched a nationwide interoperability initiative to connect hospitals, primary care providers, and pharmacies through a unified EHR framework that uses HL7 FHIR standards.

Key Takeaways: Role of interoperability in data-sharing efficiency, strategies for overcoming fragmented IT landscapes.

Case Study #4: NHS Digital's Cybersecurity and Privacy Framework

Summary: NHS Digital established a rigorous cybersecurity and privacy governance framework to protect patient data across Digital Health applications, including telemedicine and AI-driven tools.

Key Takeaways: This session will discuss best practices for data security, ensure compliance with GDPR and HIPAA, and mitigate the risks of data breaches.

Case Study #5: Mount Sinai Health System's Digital Training Academy

Summary: Mount Sinai established a Digital Health Training Academy to enhance the skills of clinicians and staff in telehealth best practices, AI-driven diagnostics, and EHR-integrated decision support tools.

Key Takeaways: The importance of ongoing education, strategies for engaging frontline staff, and methods for reducing resistance to change.

Case Study #6: Geisinger Health's RPM Success Metrics

Summary: Geisinger Health has implemented a remote patient monitoring (RPM) program for heart failure patients, tracking key performance indicators (KPIs) such as reduced readmissions and improved medication adherence. Data-driven insights have led to a permanent expansion of the program.

Key Takeaways: Measure clinical and operational impact, define key performance indicators (KPIs), and scale successful Digital Health interventions.

Practical Exercises

Exercise #1: Conducting a Digital Health Readiness Assessment Choose a healthcare setting (e.g., a large hospital, a rural clinic, or a primary care practice); identify three major clinical or operational challenges that Digital Medicine could help address; assess infrastructure readiness (EHR integration, network stability), workforce digital literacy, and financial feasibility; draft a readiness report highlighting potential barriers and enablers.

Reflection Question: What are the most significant gaps in the organization's readiness, and how could they be addressed?

Exercise #2: Evaluating a Digital Health Tool for Clinical Use Select a Digital Health tool (e.g., an AI-driven diagnostic platform, a telemedicine solution, or a wearable health device); evaluate its clinical validation, regulatory compliance, user-friendliness, and integration capabilities with existing EHR systems; compare its benefits and drawbacks relative to other available solutions.

Reflection Question: What factors would influence a clinician's decision to adopt this tool?

Exercise #3: Workflow Integration Planning Select a healthcare scenario in which a new digital tool, such as a remote patient monitoring system, is being implemented. Outline the current workflow and identify the integration points for the new technology. Detail the roles and responsibilities of clinicians, IT teams, and administrative staff. Propose a plan to optimize documentation and manage alerts.

Reflection Question: How can alert fatigue be minimized while ensuring that critical notifications are addressed?

Exercise #4: Implementing a Change Management Strategy Envision that your healthcare organization is implementing an AI-based clinical decision support tool; create a change management plan that encompasses leadership engagement, staff training, and pilot testing; suggest approaches to identify and empower "digital champions" amongst the staff.

Reflection Question: What are the most common sources of resistance to digital transformation, and how can they be mitigated?

Exercise #5: Defining Key Performance Indicators (KPIs) for Digital Health Initiatives Choose a Digital Health initiative (e.g., a telehealth program for chronic disease management); define three clinical, operational, and patient-focused KPIs to assess success; propose a strategy for data collection to monitor these KPIs over time.

Reflection Question: How can real-world data be used to refine and scale Digital Health programs?

Final Thoughts

By incorporating these case studies and practical exercises, Chap. 4 obtains a strong real-world focus, making it more actionable for healthcare professionals. These additions help bridge the gap between theoretical frameworks and real-world implementation, providing structured learning opportunities that enhance engagement and practical application.

Suggested Reading

1. Greenhalgh T, Wherton J, Papoutsi C, Lynch J, Hughes G, A'Court C, Hinder S, Fahy N, Procter R, Shaw S. Beyond adoption: a new framework for theorizing and evaluating nonadoption, abandonment, and challenges to the scale-up, spread, and sustainability of health and care technologies. J Med Internet Res. 2017;19(11):e367.
2. Chaet D, Clearfield R, Sabin JE, Skimming K. Ethical practice in telehealth and telemedicine. J Gen Intern Med. 2017;32(10):1136–40.
3. Bodenheimer T, Sinsky C. From triple to quadruple aim: care of the patient requires care of the provider. Ann Fam Med. 2014;12(6):573–6.
4. Meskó B, Győrffy Z. Robotic health: a glimpse into the future. Int J Med Robot Comput Assist Surg. 2020;16(1):e2066.
5. Shaw J, McNeil K, Calvert J, et al. The doctor is online—a systematic review of academic research on teleconsultation: the patient experience. J Telemed Telecare. 2017;23(2):155–65.
6. Carayon P, Wooldridge A, Hose B-Z, Eithun B, Fackler J. Challenges in health IT usability and the end-user's perspective. BMJ Qual Saf. 2018;27(11):970–3.
7. Kruse CS, Soma M, Pulluri D, Nemali NT, Brooks M. The effectiveness of telemedicine in the management of chronic heart disease—a systematic review. JRSM Open. 2017;8(3):2054270416681747.
8. Gopal G, Gopal A. Change management approaches for telehealth integration in healthcare settings. BMJ Innov. 2020;6(3):78–82.
9. Rowe TA, Patel A. Implementing telemedicine in response to COVID-19 in geriatric care: a pragmatic approach. Geriatrics. 2020;5(4):88.
10. Obermeyer Z, Emanuel EJ. Predicting the future—big data, machine learning, and clinical medicine. N Engl J Med. 2016;375(13):1216–9.
11. Topol E. Deep medicine: how artificial intelligence can make healthcare human again. Basic Books; 2019.
12. Wachter RM. The digital doctor: hope, hype, and harm at the dawn of medicine's computer age. McGraw-Hill Education; 2015.
13. Meskó B. The role of artificial intelligence in precision medicine. Expert Rev Precis Med Drug Dev. 2017;2(5):239–41.
14. Coiera E. The importance of trust in digital health. BMJ Qual Saf. 2015;24(4):244–5.
15. Rivas H, Wac K, editors. Digital health: scaling healthcare to the world. Springer; 2018.
16. Mandl KD, Kohane IS. A learning health system for better healthcare. N Engl J Med. 2017;376(13):1218–9.
17. Bates DW, Sheikh A. The future of health information technology in the patient-centered medical home. Health Aff. 2018;37(1):204–10.
18. Haux R. Health informatics and systems thinking. Int J Med Inform. 2020;144:104296.
19. Gulshan V, Peng L, Coram M, Stumpe MC, Wu D, Narayanaswamy A, Venugopalan S, Widner K, Madams T, Cuadros J, Kim R, Raman R, Nelson PC, Mega JL, Webster DR. Developing and validating a deep learning algorithm for detection of diabetic retinopathy in retinal fundus photographs. JAMA. 2016;316(22):2402–10.
20. Berwick DM, Nolan TW, Whittington J. The triple aim: care, health, and cost. Health Aff. 2008;27(3):759–69.
21. Meskó B, Drobni Z, Bényei É, Gergely B, Győrffy Z. Digital health is a cultural transformation of traditional healthcare. Mhealth. 2017;3:38. https://doi.org/10.21037/mhealth.2017.08.07.
22. Topol EJ. High-performance medicine: the convergence of human and artificial intelligence. Nat Med. 2019;25(1):44–56. https://doi.org/10.1038/s41591-018-0300-7.
23. Jiang F, Jiang Y, Zhi H, et al. Artificial intelligence in healthcare: past, present and future. Stroke Vasc Neurol. 2017;2(4):230–43. https://doi.org/10.1136/svn-2017-000101.
24. World Health Organization. WHO guideline: recommendations on digital interventions for health system strengthening [Internet]. 2019. Available online: https://www.who.int/publications/i/item/9789241550505

25. World Health Organization. Ethics and governance of artificial intelligence for health: WHO guidance [Internet] 2021. Available online: https://www.who.int/publications/i/item/9789240029200
26. World Health Organization. Consolidated telemedicine implementation guide [Internet]. 2022. Available online: https://www.who.int/publications/i/item/9789240059184
27. Kruse CS, Karem P, Shifflett K, et al. Evaluating barriers to adopting telemedicine worldwide: a systematic review. J Telemed Telecare. 2018;24(1):4–12. https://doi.org/10.1177/1357633X16674087.
28. Centers for Disease Control and Prevention. Using telehealth to expand access to essential health services during the COVID-19 pandemic [Internet]. 2020. Available online: https://www.cdc.gov/coronavirus/2019-ncov/hcp/telehealth.html
29. Koonin LM, Hoots B, Tsang CA, et al. Trends in the use of telehealth during the emergence of the COVID-19 pandemic — United States, January–March 2020. MMWR Morb Mortal Wkly Rep. 2020;69(43):1595–9. https://doi.org/10.15585/mmwr.mm6943a3.
30. Dicuonzo G, Galeone G, Shini M, Massari A. Towards the use of big data in healthcare: a literature review. Healthcare (Basel). 2022;10(7):1232. https://doi.org/10.3390/healthcare10071232.
31. Murdoch TB, Detsky AS. The inevitable application of big data to health care. JAMA. 2013;309(13):1351–2. https://doi.org/10.1001/jama.2013.393.
32. Howe JL, Adams KT, Hettinger AZ, et al. Electronic health record usability issues and potential contribution to patient harm. JAMA. 2018;319(12):1276–8. https://doi.org/10.1001/jama.2018.1171.
33. Istituto Superiore di Sanità. Rapporto ISS COVID-19 n. 12/2020: Indicazioni ad interim per servizi assistenziali di telemedicina durante l'emergenza sanitaria COVID-19 [Internet]. 2020. Available online: https://www.iss.it/documents/20126/0/Rapporto+ISS+COVID-19+n.+12+telemedicina.pdf
34. European Medicines Agency. HMA-EMA Joint Big Data Taskforce – summary report [Internet]. 2019. Available online: https://www.ema.europa.eu/documents/minutes/hma/ema-joint-task-force-big-data-summary-report_en.pdf
35. National Institutes of Health. NIH Strategic Plan for Data Science [Internet] 2018. Available online: https://datascience.nih.gov/sites/default/files/NIH_Strategic_Plan_for_Data_Science_Final_508.pdf
36. Health Education England. The Topol Review: Preparing the healthcare workforce to deliver the digital future [Internet]. 2019. Available online: https://topol.hee.nhs.uk/
37. European Commission. White Paper on Artificial Intelligence: a European approach to excellence and trust [Internet]. 2020. Available online: https://ec.europa.eu/newsroom/dae/document.cfm?doc_id=68342
38. Coravos A, Khozin S, Mandl KD. Developing and adopting safe and effective digital biomarkers to improve patient outcomes. npj Digit Med. 2019;2:14. https://doi.org/10.1038/s41746-019-0090-4.
39. Bashshur RL, Shannon GW, Smith BR, et al. The empirical foundations of telemedicine interventions for chronic disease management. Telemed J E Health. 2014;20(9):769–800. https://doi.org/10.1089/tmj.2014.9981.
40. Rajkomar A, Dean J, Kohane IS. Machine learning in medicine. N Engl J Med. 2019;380(14):1347–58. https://doi.org/10.1056/NEJMra1814259.
41. World Health Organization. WHO guideline: recommendations on digital interventions for health system strengthening. Geneva: World Health Organization; 2019.
42. World Health Organization. Consolidated telemedicine implementation guide. World Health. 2022; Organization
43. World Health Organization. Ethics and governance of artificial intelligence for health: WHO guidance. World Health Organization; 2021.
44. Myrick KL, Mahar M, DeFrances CJ. Telemedicine use among physicians by physician specialty: United States, 2021. NCHS Data Brief. 2024;493:1–8. Hyattsville, MD: National Center for Health Statistics. https://doi.org/10.15620/cdc:141934.

45. European Medicines Agency. Reflection paper on the use of artificial intelligence (AI) in the medicinal product lifecycle. European Medicines Agency; 2024.
46. European Union. Regulation (EU) 2016/679 of the European Parliament and of the council (general data protection regulation). Off J Eur Union. 2016;L119:1–88.
47. Istituto Superiore di Sanità. Indicazioni ad interim per servizi assistenziali di telemedicina durante l'emergenza sanitaria COVID-19 (Rapporto ISS COVID-19 n. 12/2020). Roma: Istituto Superiore di Sanità; 2020.
48. Yu KH, Beam AL, Kohane IS. Artificial intelligence in healthcare. Nat Biomed Eng. 2018;2(10):719–31. https://doi.org/10.1038/s41551-018-0305-z.
49. Schwamm LH, Pletcher S, Erskine A. AI and technology enabled clinical workflow redesign. Telemed Rep. 2024;5(1):415–20. https://doi.org/10.1089/tmr.2024.0079.
50. Ratwani RM, Reider J, Singh H. A decade of health information technology usability challenges and the path forward. JAMA. 2019;321(8):743–4. https://doi.org/10.1001/jama.2019.0161.
51. Mehta N, Pandit A. Concurrence of big data analytics and healthcare: a systematic review. Int J Med Inform. 2018;114:57–65. https://doi.org/10.1016/j.ijmedinf.2018.03.013.
52. Dash S, Shakyawar SK, Sharma M, Kaushik S. Big data in healthcare: management, analysis and future prospects. J Big Data. 2019;6:54. https://doi.org/10.1186/s40537-019-0217-0.
53. Coventry L, Branley D. Cybersecurity in healthcare: a narrative review of trends, threats and ways forward. Maturitas. 2018;113:48–52. https://doi.org/10.1016/j.maturitas.2018.04.008.
54. Topol E. Preparing the healthcare workforce to deliver the digital future (the Topol review). National Health Service, Health Education England; 2019.
55. Dorsey ER, Topol EJ. Telemedicine 2020 and the next decade. Lancet. 2020;395(10227):859. https://doi.org/10.1016/S0140-6736(20)30424-4.
56. Mandl KD, Kohane IS. A 21st-century health IT system — creating a real-world information economy. N Engl J Med. 2017;376(20):1905–7. https://doi.org/10.1056/NEJMp1700235.
57. Greenhalgh T, Wherton J, Papoutsi C, Lynch J, Hughes G, A'Court C, et al. Beyond adoption: a new framework for theorizing and evaluating nonadoption, abandonment, and challenges to the scale-up, spread, and sustainability of health and care technologies. J Med Internet Res. 2017;19(11):e367. https://doi.org/10.2196/jmir.8775.
58. World Health Organization. Global strategy on digital health 2020–2025. World Health Organization; 2021.

Overcoming Barriers to Digital Medicine Adoption

5

Common Barriers to Adoption

The adoption of Digital Medicine presents complexities that are far from straightforward. Challenges may manifest at every level, ranging from the acquisition of adequate resources to obtaining buy-in from stakeholders. This section thoroughly explores these barriers, critically examining financial constraints, cultural resistance, and organizational hurdles.

Financial and Resource Constraints

For numerous healthcare organizations, the financial burden associated with the adoption of digital solutions continues to present a substantial constraint. The implementation of telehealth infrastructure, wearable devices, AI-assisted diagnostics, and comprehensive staff training typically necessitates considerable upfront investment. This challenge is exacerbated when the anticipated benefits—such as reductions in hospital admissions or enhancements in chronic disease management—are expected to materialize only over time, often years subsequent to implementation. This temporal disparity between investment and outcomes can dissuade decision-makers, particularly within publicly funded systems where annual budgets predominate planning cycles.

Structural issues in reimbursement further complicate the situation. Numerous digital interventions—such as app-based therapy management, digital therapeutics, or remote patient monitoring—lack standardized billing codes. This results in ambiguity regarding cost coverage, with providers frequently absorbing expenses or depending on patients' out-of-pocket contributions. Public payers may impose restrictive prerequisites for coverage, confining reimbursement to specific use cases or pilot programs, thereby engendering fragmentation and uncertainty.

A. Cesario et al., *Digital Medicine Starter Guide*,
https://doi.org/10.1007/978-3-032-01272-2_5

These difficulties are especially prominent in welfare-based healthcare systems like Italy's, where the commitment to universal access must continuously be reconciled with the evolving demands of innovation. However, significant developments are underway. A notable instance is the establishment of the Intergruppo Parlamentare sulle Terapie Digitali *(Inter-Parliamentary Group on Digital Health and Digital Therapeutics)*, a cross-party parliamentary working group dedicated to advancing legislation and policy frameworks for digital therapeutics. The group receives active support from a Comitato Tecnico Scientifico *(Scientific & Technical Committee)*, comprised of subject-matter experts from clinical, regulatory, technological, and economic domains, who contribute to defining standards of evidence and policy priorities.

One of the group's principal contributions has been the promotion of Disegno di Legge 1208-C, which aspires to formally introduce digital therapies into the national health framework, thereby enabling their inclusion among reimbursable services. The legislation delineates criteria for clinical validation, regulatory oversight, and eventual integration into the Livelli Essenziali di Assistenza - LEA *(Essential Levels of Care)*—the set of healthcare services guaranteed to all citizens under the Italian National Health Service (SSN). This initiative represents a pivotal advancement toward aligning innovation with institutional sustainability, transitioning from pilot projects to structured and equitable adoption.

Meanwhile, numerous healthcare providers are adopting phased implementation strategies to mitigate risk. For example, a hospital may initiate a remote monitoring program targeting a particular patient population—such as individuals with uncontrolled hypertension—and assess short-term outcomes such as reduced emergency visits or improved medication adherence. These results can subsequently justify broader adoption, attract external funding, or stimulate interest from value-based care initiatives. As previously mentioned and further elaborated in the subsequent chapter, such strategies enable organizations to effectively manage uncertainty while cultivating a repository of real-world evidence.

Furthermore, public–private collaborations are increasingly significant. Technology firms may co-finance implementation studies or offer in-kind support to validate their products within clinical settings. Nonprofit foundations and research consortia often act as facilitators, bridging the gap between innovation and public interest. Concurrently, the ongoing shift toward outcome-oriented healthcare financing creates opportunities for digital tools that demonstrably enhance patient outcomes to gain recognition—and reimbursement—as integral components of care.

In this evolving ecosystem, financial and resource constraints remain tangible; however, they are not insurmountable. Legislative endeavors such as Disegno di Legge 1208-C in Italy, in conjunction with strategic partnerships and value-based pilot programs, are gradually transforming the landscape toward a more sustainable model—one in which digital medicine is no longer regarded as an experimental adjunct, but rather as a reimbursable, evidence-based pillar of contemporary healthcare.

Cultural and Organizational Resistance

Digital transformation signifies not only a technological change but also a substantial cultural shift. Resistance frequently emerges from apprehension, skepticism, or ambiguity. Clinicians may express concern that artificial intelligence (AI) or automation will replace their expertise, while administrators may question the efficacy of unverified tools. Patients might possess apprehensions regarding the lack of human interaction in digitally mediated care.

The potential disruption to workflows exacerbates resistance. As elaborated in Chap. 4, the introduction of AI-driven alerts or telemedicine platforms may necessitate a reevaluation of documentation processes or a redistribution of responsibilities among clinical teams.

Overcoming these cultural barriers requires transparent communication and collaborative planning. Leadership should actively involve stakeholders—clinicians, nurses, and administrative personnel—during the planning phase, ensuring that their perspectives are incorporated into the design of workflows. Training programs must extend beyond technical instruction to address concerns related to role displacement, highlighting how digital tools augment, rather than replace, clinical expertise.

For instance, organizations can establish peer mentorship programs in which "digital champions" support their colleagues in adapting to new workflows, thereby fostering confidence and trust. Periodic updates on the measurable benefits of digital tools, such as improved patient outcomes or reduced workloads, can further encourage stakeholder buy-in.

Data Privacy and Security

Chapters 2 and 3 underscore the premise that patient trust is crucial to Digital Medicine. Such trust may swiftly diminish in the absence of robust safeguards for data privacy and security. This section delineates the dual challenges of regulatory compliance and cybersecurity.

Regulatory Complexities

Navigating the complex framework of regulations that govern digital medicine constitutes a substantial challenge. Healthcare organizations frequently operate within overlapping frameworks, including HIPAA (United States), GDPR (European Union), and various regional guidelines, each with its own distinct requirements for data management and breach notification. The rapid evolution of legislation further complicates this environment. For instance, the EU AI Act introduces new compliance challenges for organizations that utilize artificial intelligence in clinical settings.

To effectively address these challenges, healthcare providers must prioritize compliance audits and consistently review their data collection and sharing practices to ensure alignment with current standards. Engaging legal experts who specialize in healthcare and technology represents a crucial step, particularly for organizations operating across multiple jurisdictions. Furthermore, adopting a data minimization approach—collecting only the information necessary for clinical care or analytics—serves to mitigate exposure to privacy risks.

Cybersecurity Threats

The expanding digital footprints of healthcare organizations render these entities appealing targets for cyberattacks. Incidents such as ransomware attacks or data breaches possess the potential to disrupt clinical workflows, compromise patient privacy, and tarnish the reputations of organizations. As emphasized in Chap. 3, these risks constitute not merely technical challenges; they also undermine patient confidence in digital tools.

Organizations must implement robust IT policies to safeguard against cybersecurity threats. This encompasses the mandatory use of multi-factor authentication, the encryption of data both during transit and at rest, and the securing of APIs employed for data exchange. Continuous monitoring alongside intrusion detection systems can aid in the identification and mitigation of threats in real time. Ultimately, incident response plans should be established, delineating clear steps for containment, recovery, and communication.

Digital Divide, Patients, and Health Operators Literacy

As explored in Chap. 3, the digital divide remains one of the most persistent challenges to the equitable deployment of Digital Medicine. While technological innovation has brought forward powerful tools for care delivery, it has also laid bare critical disparities in access, digital literacy, and technological readiness—especially among vulnerable populations. These disparities not only limit the effectiveness of digital interventions but also risk reinforcing pre-existing health inequalities.

In health systems like Italy's Servizio Sanitario Nazionale (SSN), where universality and subsidiarity are foundational principles, addressing the digital divide is not merely a technical task—it is an ethical imperative. Ensuring that no patient is left behind in the digital transition requires a systemic, multi-stakeholder response.

Access to Technology

Reliable access to technology is often assumed, but in practice, it remains a barrier for many. In rural or underserved areas, broadband infrastructure may be insufficient for video consultations or real-time data transmission from connected devices.

Low-income households may lack access to smartphones, tablets, or even stable internet connectivity.

A patient living in a small mountain town in central Italy, for instance, may have a smartphone but no reliable signal or broadband service. Scheduling a teleconsultation with a specialist located in a regional hub may become impractical, forcing the patient to rely on infrequent and often costly in-person visits. This dynamic, if unaddressed, undermines the potential of Digital Medicine to deliver more convenient and proactive care.

Strategies to Bridge Access Gaps

Bridging the digital divide demands both structural reforms and immediate, actionable solutions. Long-term investments in broadband expansion and digital infrastructure are essential—but in the meantime, healthcare organizations can adopt adaptive strategies such as loaner devices and offline-capable applications, which allow care delivery to reach patients regardless of their connectivity status or digital ownership.

Loaner Devices

Loaner programs represent a pragmatic way to ensure that patients lacking access to digital tools can still benefit from remote monitoring or teleconsultation services. By providing pre-configured smartphones, tablets, or wearables on a temporary basis, healthcare organizations can remove a significant access barrier without imposing direct financial burdens on patients.

For example, an Italian local health authority (ASL) piloting a home monitoring program for COPD patients might offer a kit consisting of a pulse oximeter and a tablet with preloaded software. Once the treatment period concludes, the kit is returned and refurbished for the next patient. This model supports both clinical continuity and economic sustainability.

Key Considerations for Loaner Programs

1. Ease of Setup: Devices must be plug-and-play, with intuitive interfaces and minimal configuration requirements. Clear, language-accessible instructions—possibly delivered during hospital discharge—can support rapid onboarding.
2. Ongoing Support: A help desk or hotline, possibly staffed by community volunteers or digital health navigators, can address troubleshooting and promote continued engagement.
3. Sustainability and Partnerships: Collaborations with device manufacturers, social cooperatives, or regional digital health initiatives (such as those funded under the PNRR Missione 6 in Italy) can offset costs and ensure scalability.

Offline Applications

In parallel, offline-capable apps offer a crucial solution for patients with unreliable or intermittent Internet access. These tools allow patients to log vital signs, receive educational content, and follow treatment instructions without needing constant connectivity. Once a connection becomes available—via public Wi-Fi or mobile hotspot—data is securely synced with healthcare systems.

A maternal health app deployed in Calabria or Sardinia, for instance, could track prenatal checklists and deliver culturally adapted content even in areas with patchy coverage. Upon visiting a local clinic, the app would automatically upload stored information to the patient's digital record.

Advantages of Offline Applications

- Resilience in underserved areas or economically disadvantaged neighborhoods.
- Security, with sensitive data stored locally until transmission is possible.
- Inclusivity, allowing equal access regardless of location or socioeconomic background.

Combining Strategies for Maximum Impact

The most effective approaches combine both strategies. A healthcare provider might supply a tablet with a pre-installed offline telehealth app, ensuring the patient has both the device and a way to use it even in connectivity-poor environments. Such integrative models help dismantle multiple barriers simultaneously, extending the benefits of digital medicine across population groups that are often overlooked.

These approaches are increasingly being adopted in regional pilots across Italy, often under the guidance of Digital Health Units (UVD) or in collaboration with local municipalities. Their success depends not only on the technology itself, but on how it is delivered, supported, and sustained over time.

Health Literacy and Usability

Even when access is secured, digital literacy remains a major limiting factor—not only for patients but also for healthcare professionals. Confidence in using digital tools, understanding app logic, and troubleshooting simple problems is often assumed but not guaranteed.

Older adults may struggle with device charging, notifications, or app syncing. Language barriers can also interfere with comprehension, particularly in tools that lack multilingual or culturally tailored support. Similarly, clinicians may feel unprepared to integrate digital workflows into their routines, especially if training is insufficient or poorly timed.

Strategies for Enhancing Digital Literacy and Usability

- User-Centered Design: Tools must be designed with real users in mind—featuring large buttons, clear visual cues, and accessible language. This applies to both patient-facing and clinician-facing interfaces.

- Multilingual and Cultural Adaptation: Especially relevant in Italy, where growing migrant populations demand interfaces that reflect linguistic and cultural diversity.
- Community-Based Outreach: Partnering with public libraries, parishes, and civic associations to offer digital health literacy workshops can demystify the tools and build trust—both with patients and providers.
- Training for Healthcare Professionals: Including digital literacy modules in continuing education (ECM) programs or in the implementation plans of new digital services, as encouraged by national digital health strategies.

In summary, tackling the digital divide requires more than technology—it requires infrastructure, policy, and inclusive design. And it requires a commitment to seeing access, literacy, and usability not as peripheral issues, but as central determinants of whether digital medicine fulfills its promise of health equity. In systems like the SSN, where universalism is a foundational value, this is not just a strategic concern. It is a matter of public trust.

Reimbursement and Legal Ambiguities

As discussed in Chap. 2, Digital Medicine holds the potential to transform healthcare delivery by improving access, continuity of care, and clinical outcomes. However, outdated reimbursement mechanisms and unresolved legal frameworks continue to act as significant barriers. These challenges not only discourage innovation but also often prevent healthcare providers from scaling effective digital interventions.

The situation varies significantly between countries, depending on how healthcare is funded, regulated, and organized. In insurance-driven systems like the United States, reimbursement is tightly linked to billing codes and payer-specific contracts, making innovation possible but frequently fragmented. In contrast, universalist models such as Italy's Servizio Sanitario Nazionale (SSN) must balance innovation with equity and budgetary oversight, often moving more slowly but within a framework of public accountability.

Payment Models for Digital Care

Most traditional payment models were not designed with digital services in mind. As a result, healthcare organizations attempting to implement tools like remote patient monitoring (RPM), AI-driven diagnostics, or app-based disease management often face structural challenges such as:

- Lack of Billing Codes: Many digital services are not yet formally codified in national reimbursement systems, making them difficult to fund through standard procedures.

- Out-of-Pocket Costs: When coverage is absent or partial, patients are often required to pay for digital tools themselves—raising concerns about affordability and access.
- Inconsistent Reimbursement Policies: Especially in decentralized systems, reimbursement for telehealth and digital interventions may vary between regions, insurers, or clinical contexts, generating uncertainty for both providers and innovators.

In Italy, for example, while several regional authorities have initiated pilot programs for telemonitoring and digital therapeutics, national-level reimbursement remains under development. The recent Disegno di Legge 1208-C on digital therapies marks a step forward by proposing the introduction of structured pathways for validation and reimbursement of these tools within the LEA *(Essential Levels of Care)*. However, until such provisions are institutionalized, many providers remain hesitant to scale these services beyond small trials.

By contrast, Germany's DiGA framework offers an advanced model of reimbursement for certified digital health applications. Once an app passes clinical and technical evaluation under BfArM (Federal Institute for Drugs and Medical Devices), it can be listed and prescribed with full reimbursement by statutory health insurers. The UK's NHS, while less centralized in its digital health reimbursement pathways, has introduced innovation accelerators and dedicated evaluation units (e.g., NICE Evidence Standards Framework) to integrate cost-effectiveness into digital care adoption.

Examples and Strategies

- Value-Based Care Contracts: Hospitals implementing RPM for chronic heart failure have secured shared-savings agreements with insurers by demonstrating reduced readmission rates. This model has gained traction in the United States, where financial risk-sharing is embedded in Medicare's ACOs (Accountable Care Organizations). In Italy, regional experiments in Lombardy and Emilia-Romagna have begun to explore similar models, though not yet at scale.
- Pilot Programs: Demonstration projects remain a key strategy to bridge the gap between innovation and reimbursement. For example, several Italian ASLs (Local Health Authorities) have partnered with universities and tech firms to trial digital solutions for diabetes or COPD, collecting real-world data that could support future reimbursement claims. Similarly, in France, the Article 51 framework enables experimentation with new models of care, including digital health, with temporary funding pending formal inclusion in the national scheme.

Cross-Border Telemedicine

The capacity of telemedicine to transcend geographic boundaries presents promising opportunities—particularly for specialist consultations and remote second opinions—while simultaneously generating intricate legal and regulatory challenges. These challenges encompass:

1. *Licensing and Jurisdiction*: A provider licensed in one country may not possess the requisite authorization to practice in another, thus raising legal issues pertaining to the provision of virtual care across borders.
2. *Data Privacy*: Regulations such as the European Union's General Data Protection Regulation (GDPR) establish stringent rules governing the processing of personal health data, particularly when providers operate from outside the EU.
3. *Liability and Legal Redress*: The uncertainty regarding which jurisdiction's laws apply in instances of medical error or miscommunication may dissuade providers from offering cross-border digital care.

In the European Union, certain measures have been enacted to promote regulatory convergence—for instance, the eHealth Digital Service Infrastructure (eHDSI) facilitates the exchange of ePrescriptions and Patient Summaries among member states. Nevertheless, comprehensive telemedicine frameworks continue to exhibit fragmentation. Italy, for instance, has promulgated national telemedicine guidelines (2020), yet these guidelines predominantly apply within its own national boundaries. Currently, no formal mechanisms exist to acknowledge non-Italian licenses for the provision of care to Italian residents via digital platforms.

Conversely, systems such as that of the United States have sought to address the aforementioned challenges through reciprocal licensing compacts (e.g., Interstate Medical Licensure Compact), although these arrangements remain dependent on state-specific regulations. On a global scale, agencies such as the World Health Organization (WHO) and the Organisation for Economic Co-operation and Development (OECD) have advocated for the harmonization of telemedicine practices; however, legally binding frameworks are still absent.

Strategies for Cross-Border Solutions

Reciprocal Licensing Agreements: The mutual recognition of medical qualifications—such as those pursued within the European Union and pursuant to bilateral treaties—can facilitate legal clarity and enable secure cross-border teleconsultations.

Harmonized Regulations: International endeavors to standardize digital health terminology, consent procedures, and care protocols can diminish legal uncertainty and promote trust. Organizations such as the World Health Organization (WHO) and the International Organization for Standardization (ISO) are active in this domain but frequently lack enforcement authority.

Liability Protocols: Institutions providing cross-border care must establish clear internal protocols, contractual disclaimers, and insurance policies delineating the applicable jurisdiction's laws—especially in the context of medico-legal disputes.

In summary, reimbursement and legal frameworks continue to function as the "slow gears" in the apparatus of Digital Medicine. Their evolution—whether

Table 5.1 Digital Health Reimbursement and regulatory Comparison

Country/ system	Digital health reimbursement framework	Approval and evaluation process	Legal/regulatory considerations
Italy (SSN)	In development—DDL 1208-C aims to integrate Digital Therapeutics (DTx) into LEA; some regional pilots ongoing	To be defined; current evaluations are regional and pilot-based	National telemedicine guidelines; GDPR applies; no cross-border licensing in place
Germany (DiGA)	DiGA fast track: Certified apps can be reimbursed by statutory insurers after BfArM approval	Formal process through BfArM including clinical benefit and data security evaluation	Clear data and privacy standards; embedded in EU law; BfArM manages compliance
France (Article 51)	Article 51 experiments enable temporary funding for digital health pilots; potential national adoption	Regional Health Agencies (ARS) evaluate outcomes; coordinated by Ministry of Health	Must comply with CNIL and EU regulations; experimentation governed by article 51
United Kingdom (NHS)	Innovation accelerators and NICE evidence framework guide adoption; no centralized reimbursement path	Evidence-based review via NICE; emphasis on cost-effectiveness and real-world impact	Mixed framework: UK GDPR; local trusts manage implementation
United States (Medicare/ private)	CPT codes for telehealth and some RPM; reimbursement varies widely by payer and state	FDA clearance for some tools; reimbursement depends on coding and payer policy	HIPAA-compliant systems required; licensing and liability governed by state laws

through national legislation such as Disegno di Legge 1208-C in Italy, or transnational standards emerging within the European Union—is crucial to ensuring that innovation progresses not only swiftly but also safely, sustainably, and equitably. Refer for a synthesis to Table 5.1.

Cultivating Digital Literacy and Trust

As noted in Chaps. 1 and 4, the success of Digital Medicine relies on building confidence and competence among clinicians and patients. Trust and education are essential for sustained engagement with digital tools.

Training Clinicians and Administrators

Healthcare professionals often face steep learning curves when integrating new technologies into their workflows. In addition to technical know-how, they must develop confidence in interpreting data from AI systems or wearable devices.

Strategies for Building Expertise

Continuous Education: Integrate Digital Health training into medical school curricula and ongoing certification programs.

Mentorship Programs: Appoint 'digital champions" within healthcare teams to offer guidance and promote peer-to-peer learning.

Workload Adjustments: Allocate time for clinicians to become acquainted with new systems, ensuring that the adoption of technology does not worsen burnout.

Engaging Patients and Caregivers

Patients' trust in digital tools depends on transparency, ease of use, and perceived benefits. For example, a patient managing asthma with a smart inhaler might abandon it if they feel their data isn't secure or the device's interface is unintuitive.

Strategies for Patient Engagement

Transparent Data Practices: Clarify how patient data is collected, stored, and utilized. Offering opt-in controls fosters trust.

Gamification: Incorporating motivational elements, such as earning badges for regular use, helps keep patients engaged over time.

Feedback Mechanisms: Patients should be able to share concerns or suggestions for improving digital tools, fostering collaboration and accountability.

Looking Ahead

As the healthcare ecosystem undergoes its digital transformation, it is vital to tackle barriers such as financial constraints, privacy concerns, and skill gaps. Successful organizations will prioritize patient-centric solutions, align their strategies with evolving regulations, and promote digital literacy across all stakeholder groups. By doing so, they can unlock Digital Medicine's potential to create a more equitable, efficient, and compassionate healthcare system.

Key Takeaways

Barriers are multifaceted: address financial, cultural, and infrastructural challenges with bespoke strategies.

Trust is paramount: Open communication and patient-centered design cultivate trust among stakeholders.

Education and Outreach Are Essential: Continuous training helps clinicians and patients stay engaged and confident in using digital tools.

Policy Evolution: Modernize reimbursement and legal frameworks to align with the realities of Digital Healthcare.

Equity and Accessibility: Bridging digital divides ensures that no patient or provider is left behind during this transformation.

Case Studies and Practical Exercises

Case Studies

Case Study #1: Remote Patient Monitoring (RPM) for Chronic Conditions—Cleveland Clinic

Summary: Cleveland Clinic piloted an RPM program for chronic disease management using a phased approach. The program initially focused on a small patient cohort, demonstrating improved health outcomes and cost reductions. Positive results led to broader implementation with financial support from payers.

Key Takeaways: Phased implementation, securing financial sustainability through reimbursement, demonstrating ROI.

Case Study #2: Mayo Clinic's AI Integration Strategy

Summary: Mayo Clinic implemented an AI-based clinical decision support tool but faced initial resistance from physicians concerned about automation replacing human expertise. To build trust, the institution launched clinician-led AI training programs and involved medical staff in system customization.

Key Takeaways: Importance of stakeholder engagement, clinician-led training, aligning digital tools with existing workflows.

Case Study #3: GDPR Compliance in Telemedicine—France's Doctolib

Summary: Doctolib, a major European telemedicine provider, navigated stringent GDPR regulations by adopting a patient-first data privacy approach, including transparent consent mechanisms and encrypted data storage.

Key Takeaways: Data protection compliance, transparency in patient data handling, and the importance of engaging legal experts.

Case Study #4: Ransomware Attack on a Healthcare Network—Universal Health Services (UHS)

Summary: UHS suffered a major ransomware attack that disrupted hospital operations for weeks. The organization responded by strengthening multi-factor authentication, implementing real-time cybersecurity monitoring, and enhancing staff training on phishing awareness.

Key Takeaways: Proactive cybersecurity measures, multi-layered security approaches, importance of staff training.

Case Study #5: Loaner Devices for Digital Health Access—Federally Qualified Health Centers (FQHCs)

Summary: Several FQHCs in the U.S. introduced a loaner tablet program for low-income patients, enabling them to participate in telehealth visits and chronic disease management programs. The initiative was supported by federal funding and private partnerships.

Key Takeaways: Bridging digital gaps, leveraging public–private funding, increasing accessibility in underserved communities.

Case Study #6: mHealth App for Elderly Patients—Singapore's Healthy365
Summary: Singapore's Ministry of Health developed Healthy365, a user-friendly mHealth app designed with large buttons, simple navigation, and multilingual support to cater to older adults. Adoption increased significantly due to a community outreach campaign.

Key Takeaways: Importance of intuitive design, multilingual support, user engagement through community initiatives.

Case Study #7: Value-Based Reimbursement for Digital Therapeutics—Germany's DiGA Program
Summary: Germany introduced the DiGA (Digital Health Applications) program, allowing doctors to prescribe clinically validated digital therapeutics covered by insurance. This model facilitated access to digital tools and provided a reimbursement framework.

Key Takeaways: Role of government policies in supporting Digital Medicine, value-based reimbursement models, ensuring long-term funding sustainability.

Case Study #8: Cross-Border eHealth Collaboration—Estonia and Finland
Summary: Estonia and Finland developed a cross-border ePrescription service, allowing citizens to retrieve medications in either country. This initiative required harmonizing regulatory frameworks and data exchange protocols.

Key Takeaways: Harmonization of telemedicine regulations, international interoperability challenges, legal and policy alignment.

Case Study #9: NHS Digital Academy—Upskilling Healthcare Professionals
Summary: The UK's NHS Digital Academy offers structured training in Digital Health for healthcare professionals, equipping them with knowledge on AI, telehealth, and EHR integration. This initiative has remarkably boosted digital adoption rates.

Key Takeaways: Structured Digital Health training, empowering clinicians, ongoing professional development.

Case Study #10: Gamification for Patient Engagement—Omada Health
Summary: Omada Health developed a digital diabetes prevention program that incorporates gamification and behavioral incentives. This program has improved patient adherence and long-term engagement.

Key Takeaways: Behavioral science in Digital Health adoption, gamification strategies, enhancing patient motivation.

Practical Exercises

Exercise #1: Overcoming Financial Barriers
Task: Assume you are a member of a hospital's digital transformation team tasked with implementing remote patient monitoring for heart failure patients. Develop a

financial plan that outlines the phased implementation, potential funding sources (e.g., grants, insurance partnerships), and projected ROI.

Reflection Question: How can you justify the long-term value of Digital Medicine to hospital administrators?

Exercise #2: Managing Cultural Resistance to Digital Health Tools
Task: Envision that your hospital is implementing an AI-based decision-support tool. Identify the main concerns of various stakeholders (physicians, nurses, patients, administrators) and propose a.

Reflection Question: How can Digital Health leaders build trust among clinicians and ensure that technology complements, rather than replaces, their expertise?

Exercise #3: Developing a Data Security and Compliance Strategy
Task: Select a Digital Health tool (e.g., a telemedicine platform or an AI-driven diagnostic system); evaluate its regulatory requirements (e.g., GDPR, HIPAA); and devise a compliance and cybersecurity strategy to protect patient data.

Reflection Question: How can healthcare organizations balance data accessibility with stringent privacy requirements?

Exercise #4: Bridging the Digital Divide
Task: Develop a proposal for a digital inclusion program that ensures underserved communities can access telemedicine services; consider solutions such as loaner devices, community training programs, and offline applications.

Reflection Question: What immediate and long-term strategies can healthcare organizations implement to address Digital Health inequities?

Exercise #5: Creating a Sustainable Reimbursement Model for Digital Health
Task: Assume you are advising a national health system on how to integrate digital therapeutics into standard care; outline a reimbursement framework that includes payer partnerships, evidence-based coverage decisions, and patient access policies.

Reflection Question: What role do policymakers and insurers play in ensuring the sustainability of Digital Health adoption?

Final Thoughts

By incorporating these case studies and practical exercises, Chap. 5 offers a structured and real-world framework for addressing the most significant obstacles to the adoption of Digital Medicine. These examples enable readers to translate theory into practice, providing them with strategies to navigate financial, regulatory, cultural, and technical challenges effectively.

Suggested Reading

1. Sood SP, Mbarika VWA, Jugoo S, Dookhy R, et al. What is telemedicine? A collection of 104 peer-reviewed perspectives and theoretical underpinnings. Telemed e-Health. 2007;13(5):573–90.
2. World Health Organization. Telemedicine: opportunities and developments in member states. Report on the second global survey on eHealth. Geneva: WHO Press; 2010.
3. World Health Organization. Global diffusion of eHealth: making universal health coverage achievable. Report of the third global survey on eHealth. Geneva: WHO Press; 2016.
4. Ekeland AG, Bowes A, Flottorp S. Effectiveness of telemedicine: a systematic review of reviews. Int J Med Inform. 2010;79(11):736–71.
5. Kruse CS, Karem P, Shifflett K, Vegi L, Ravi K, Brooks M. Evaluating barriers to adopting telemedicine worldwide: a systematic review. J Telemed Telecare. 2018;24(1):4–12.
6. Dorsey ER, Topol EJ. State of telehealth. N Engl J Med. 2016;375(2):154–61.
7. Tuckson RV, Edmunds M, Hodgkins ML. Telehealth. N Engl J Med. 2017;377(16):1585–92.
8. Stanberry B. Legal and ethical aspects of telemedicine. J Telemed Telecare. 2006;12(4):166–75.
9. Langarizadeh M, Moghbeli F, Aliabadi A. Application of ethics for providing telemedicine services and information technology. Med Arch. 2017;71(5):351–5.
10. Vayena E, Haeusermann T, Adjekum A, Blasimme A. Digital health: meeting the ethical and policy challenges. Swiss Med Wkly. 2018;148:w14571.
11. Greenhalgh T, Wherton J, Papoutsi C, et al. Beyond adoption: a new framework for theorizing and evaluating non-adoption, abandonment, and challenges to the scale-up, spread, and sustainability of health and care technologies. J Med Internet Res. 2017;19(11):e367.
12. Totten AM, Womack DM, Eden KB, McDonagh MS, et al. Telehealth: Mapping the evidence for patient outcomes from systematic reviews. Technical Brief No. 26. Rockville, MD: Agency for Healthcare Research and Quality; 2016.
13. Keesara S, Jonas A, Schulman K. Covid-19 and health care's digital revolution. N Engl J Med. 2020;382(23):e82.
14. van Dyk L. A review of telehealth service implementation frameworks. Int J Environ Res Public Health. 2014;11(2):1279–98.
15. Bashshur RL, Shannon GW, Smith BR, Alverson DC. The empirical foundations of telemedicine interventions for chronic disease management. Telemed e-Health. 2014;20(9):769–800.
16. Broens THF, Huis in 't Veld RM, Vollenbroek-Hutten MM, et al. Determinants of successful telemedicine implementations: a literature study. J Telemed Telecare. 2007;13(6):303–9.
17. Kaplan B, Litewka S. Ethical challenges of telemedicine and telehealth. Camb Q Healthc Ethics. 2008;17(4):401–16.
18. Kidholm K, Ekeland AG, Jensen LK, et al. A model for assessment of telemedicine applications (MAST). Int J Technol Assess Health Care. 2012;28(1):44–51.
19. Zanaboni P, Wootton R. Adoption of telemedicine: from pilot stage to routine delivery. BMC Med Inform Decis Mak. 2012;12:1.
20. Lucas H. Information and communications technology for future health systems in developing countries. Soc Sci Med. 2008;66(10):2122–32.
21. Borges do Nascimento IJ, Abdulazeem H, Vasanthan LT, Martinez EZ, Zucoloto ML, Østengaard L, Azzopardi-Muscat N, Zapata T, Novillo-Ortiz D. Barriers and facilitators to utilizing digital health technologies by healthcare professionals. NPJ Digital Med. 2023;6(1):161. https://doi.org/10.1038/s41746-023-00899-4.
22. Kruse CS, Heinemann K. Facilitators and barriers to the adoption of telemedicine during the first year of COVID-19: systematic review. J Med Internet Res. 2022;24(1):e31752. https://doi.org/10.2196/31752.
23. Greenhalgh T, Wherton J, Papoutsi C, Lynch J, Hughes G, A'Court C, Hinder S, Fahy N, Procter R, Shaw S. Beyond adoption: a new framework for theorizing and evaluating nonadoption, abandonment, and challenges to the scale-up, spread, and sustainability of health and care technologies. J Med Internet Res. 2017;19(11):e367. https://doi.org/10.2196/jmir.8775.

24. Nittari G, Khuman R, Baldoni S, Pallotta G, Battineni G, Sirignano A, Amenta F, Ricci G. Telemedicine practice: review of the current ethical and legal challenges. Telemed e-Health. 2020;26(12):1427–37. https://doi.org/10.1089/tmj.2019.0158.
25. World Health Organization. WHO guideline: recommendations on digital interventions for health system strengthening. Geneva: World Health Organization; 2019. https://www.who.int/publications/i/item/9789241550505
26. World Health Organization. Global strategy on digital health 2020–2025. Geneva: World Health Organization; 2021. https://www.who.int/docs/default-source/documents/gs4dh-daa2a9f352b0445bafbc79ca799dce4d.pdf
27. Bokolo AJ. Exploring the adoption of telemedicine and virtual software for care of outpatients during and after COVID-19 pandemic. Ir J Med Sci. 2021;190(1):1–10. https://doi.org/10.1007/s11845-020-02299-z.
28. Bertolazzi A, Quaglia V, Bongelli R. Barriers and facilitators to health technology adoption by older adults with chronic diseases: an integrative systematic review. BMC Public Health. 2024;24(1):506. https://doi.org/10.1186/s12889-024-18036-5.
29. Kuan PX, Chan WK, Ying DKF, Abdul Rahman MA, Peariasamy KM, Lai NM, Mills NL, Anand A. Efficacy of telemedicine for the management of cardiovascular disease: a systematic review and meta-analysis. Lancet Digital Health. 2022;4(9):e676–91. https://doi.org/10.1016/S2589-7500(22)00124-8.
30. Oliveira Hashiguchi T. Bringing health care to the patient: an overview of the use of telemedicine in OECD countries (Health Working Paper No. 116). Paris: OECD Publishing; 2020. https://www.oecd.org/en/publications/bringing-health-care-to-the-patient_8e56ede7-en.html
31. Istituto Superiore di Sanità. Rapporto ISS COVID-19 n. 12/2020: Indicazioni ad interim per servizi assistenziali di telemedicina durante l'emergenza sanitaria COVID-19 (Versione del 13 aprile 2020). Roma: Istituto Superiore di Sanità; 2020. https://www.iss.it/rapporti-covid-19/-/asset_publisher/btw1J82wtYzH/content/rapporto-iss-covid-19-n.-12-2020-indicazioni-ad-interim-per-servizi-assistenziali-di-telemedicina-durante-l-emergenza-sanitaria-covid-19.-versione-del-13-aprile-2020
32. Koonin LM, Hoots B, Tsang CA, Leroy Z, Farris K, Jolly T, Antall P, McCabe B, Zelis CBR, Tong I, Harris AM. Trends in the use of telehealth during the emergence of the COVID-19 pandemic — United States, January–March 2020. MMWR Morb Mortal Wkly Rep. 2020;69(43):1595–9. https://doi.org/10.15585/mmwr.mm6943a3.
33. Topol E. The Topol review: preparing the healthcare workforce to deliver the digital future. NHS Health Education England; 2019. https://topol.hee.nhs.uk/wp-content/uploads/HEE-Topol-Review-2019.pdf
34. Smith AC, Thomas E, Snoswell CL, Haydon H, Mehrotra A, Clemensen J, Caffery LJ. Telehealth for global emergencies: implications for coronavirus disease 2019 (COVID-19). J Telemed Telecare. 2020;26(5):309–13. https://doi.org/10.1177/1357633X20916567.
35. Damschroder LJ, Aron DC, Keith RE, Kirsh SR, Alexander JA, Lowery JC. Fostering implementation of health services research findings into practice: a consolidated framework for advancing implementation science. Implement Sci. 2009;4(1):50. https://doi.org/10.1186/1748-5908-4-50.
36. American Medical Association. AMA digital Health Research: physicians' motivations and requirements for adopting digital health. Chicago: American Medical Association; 2022. https://www.ama-assn.org/system/files/ama-digital-health-study.pdf
37. U.S. Department of Health and Human Services, Office of the Assistant Secretary for Planning and Evaluation. Trends in the use of telehealth services during the COVID-19 pandemic (Issue Brief No. HP-2022-04). 2022. https://aspe.hhs.gov/sites/default/files/documents/7d6b4989431f4c70144f209622975116/household-pulse-survey-telehealth-covid-ib.pdf
38. Flodgren G, Rachas A, Farmer AJ, Inzitari M, Shepperd S. Interactive telemedicine for managing chronic diseases. Cochrane Database Syst Rev. 2015;9:CD002098. https://doi.org/10.1002/14651858.CD002098.pub2.
39. U.S. Food and Drug Administration. Digital health innovation action plan. Silver Spring, MD: U.S. FDA; 2018. https://www.fda.gov/media/106331/download

Beyond Metrics: Rethinking Value in Digital Transformation of Healthcare

6

Introduction

Digital medicine represents one of the most promising frontiers of contemporary healthcare. It brings with it immense opportunities: improved access, more accurate diagnostics, personalized care, and enhanced efficiency. There is widespread optimism across institutions, clinicians, researchers, and patients regarding the transformative potential of digital tools. However, the very speed and scale of this transformation demand a rigorous and multidimensional analysis—not to curb innovation, but to ensure that it develops in inclusive, equitable, and sustainable ways.

While the previous chapter examined the barriers to the adoption of digital medicine—technical, regulatory, cultural, and organizational—this chapter turns to a distinct but complementary perspective: the emerging risks in an increasingly digital healthcare system.

Some themes, such as the digital divide, appear in both discussions, yet here the focus shifts. Rather than asking what slows down digital medicine, we ask what could go wrong even when it is implemented. In doing so, we emphasize that technological advancement, if not critically assessed, can inadvertently deepen inequalities, fragment care, or narrow our understanding of health.

This chapter adopts a sociological perspective to unpack how value is defined, measured, and distributed in digital medicine. It explores how dominant models—such as Value-Based Healthcare—shape decisions around funding, organization, and innovation. These models, while aiming to improve efficiency and outcomes, risk prioritizing what is easily measurable at the expense of what is relational, contextual, or ethically significant. Therefore, we advocate for a plural and situated understanding of value—one that recognizes health as not only an economic concern but also a social and human right.

When discussing sustainability in healthcare, it is essential to consider not only financial viability but also social sustainability, which encompasses the system's

A. Cesario et al., *Digital Medicine Starter Guide*,
https://doi.org/10.1007/978-3-032-01272-2_6

ability to uphold dignity, equity, participation, and long-term inclusion. Digital transformation should be guided by this comprehensive vision. The objective of this chapter is not to impede progress but to facilitate it through thoughtful reflection—ensuring that innovation becomes more equitable and intelligent, as well as faster. By proactively identifying critical risks, we can more effectively shape future developments toward a digital healthcare system that genuinely benefits all, without incurring unnecessary social or economic costs.

Value Pluralism: The Evolution of Value in Healthcare—From Clinical Centrality to Systems Thinking

Value as a Social Construct: From Classical Theory to Healthcare Implications

The concept of "value" has a rich and contested genealogy in social theory. From Marx to Weber, and more recently Boltanski and Thévenot, sociologists have shown that value is never neutral or fixed, but always embedded in specific social, historical, and institutional contexts. Marx distinguished sharply between use value (what something is good for) and exchange value (what it can be traded for), highlighting how capitalist systems tend to prioritize the latter, often at the expense of human needs. Weber emphasized the role of rationalization and the emergence of bureaucratic forms of value justification, while Boltanski and Thévenot introduced the idea of "orders of worth," showing how different spheres of social life—civic, market, industrial, domestic—deploy different evaluative logics.

These theoretical insights are especially relevant in healthcare, where decisions about what matters, what should be funded, and what counts as success are far from objective. Healthcare, by its nature, intertwines technical, ethical, and relational dimensions. As such, reducing value to merely economic or technical efficiency risks marginalizing other crucial dimensions—such as equity, dignity, and human meaning.

Shifting Models of Value: From Medical Authority to Evidence and Outcomes

Historically, healthcare systems in numerous nations—encompassing both the European welfare model and the United States' pluralistic system—have developed around what may be termed the prestational model. In this paradigm, value was implicitly associated with the volume and intensity of medical procedures, as well as the central role of the physician. Within this framework, the physician occupies an unquestioned position of authority, and healthcare delivery is predominantly characterized by clinical procedures. The model is fundamentally rooted in the biomedical tradition and has been further reinforced by fee-for-service payment structures and hierarchical professional relationships. Nevertheless, this approach has frequently led to issues such as over-treatment, fragmented care, and limited patient engagement. The value of healthcare was often equated with the quantity of interventions performed, rather than the quality or effectiveness of care.

To address certain inefficiencies, the 1990s witnessed the emergence of evidence-based medicine (EBM), which aimed to realign healthcare practices around scientific rigor and standardized knowledge. EBM prioritized the integration of the highest quality research evidence with clinical expertise and patient preferences. This represented a significant transition from an exclusively expert-driven model to one that recognized the importance of data and insights at the population level. Both European healthcare systems and the United States healthcare system adopted EBM as a fundamental framework for enhancing the quality of care, despite encountering diverse implementation challenges and contextual constraints. Nonetheless, EBM also exhibited certain limitations. It frequently favoured quantitative over qualitative knowledge, and in practice, patient values were often subordinate to generalized evidence. Furthermore, EBM was ill-equipped to address issues related to multi-morbidity, complex care scenarios, and contextual factors outside the scope of randomized controlled trials.

The early 2000s witnessed another paradigmatic turn with the emergence of value-based healthcare (VBHC), most notably theorized by Michael Porter. VBHC aimed to address the growing unsustainability of healthcare systems by redefining value as "health outcomes achieved per dollar spent." In this model, improving value meant improving outcomes while reducing costs. VBHC introduced key tools such as outcome measurement, benchmarking, and bundled payments. It also encouraged a shift from volume to results, promoting transparency and accountability. Both the European Union's health policy frameworks and US healthcare reforms increasingly integrated VBHC principles, albeit shaped by differing institutional and cultural contexts.

VBHC represented a critical advancement in linking clinical results with economic responsibility. However, over time, it became evident that the model was excessively narrow. First, it tended to define outcomes in technical and biomedical terms, often neglecting patient-reported experiences, cultural factors, and social determinants of health. Second, it assumed a universal metric of value that could be standardized across diverse contexts—an assumption that conflicted with the heterogeneity of healthcare systems and patient needs. Finally, by emphasizing individual patient value ("value for the patient"), VBHC occasionally marginalized broader issues concerning equity, access, and resource allocation.

Toward Plural and Systemic Valuation: The Emergence of the Triple Value Model

In response to these criticisms, scholars and institutions began to advocate for a more pluralistic and systemic approach to value. This evolution culminated in the development of the "Triple Value" model, which distinguishes between:

1. Personal Value—delivering care that matters to the individual, aligned with their preferences, values, and circumstances;
2. Allocative Value—ensuring resources are distributed equitably and used where they can achieve the greatest impact;
3. Technical (or Use) Value—optimizing outcomes with available resources, ensuring that interventions are effective and efficient.

This model recognizes that healthcare must balance individual, systemic, and economic perspectives. It also emphasizes co-creation, shared decision-making, and community engagement, acknowledging that value cannot be solely defined by professionals or administrators.

The European Commission, in its 2019 report "Defining Value in 'Value-Based Healthcare'," explicitly endorses this shift. It argues that value in healthcare should not be confined to economic metrics or individual outcomes but must include solidarity, equity, trust, and sustainability. Meanwhile, in the United States, the public and political discourse around healthcare value tends to emphasize individual freedom, market efficiency, and personal responsibility as core principles shaping policy and reform efforts.

In this sense, the evolution of value in healthcare mirrors broader sociological insights: value is not a fixed formula but a dynamic, negotiated construct. Each shift—from the physician-centered model, to EBM, to VBHC, to triple value—reflects an attempt to correct the blind spots of its predecessor. But each also introduces new challenges. Today, in the digital age, this evolution continues: algorithms, data platforms, and AI tools bring new promises but also risks of hyper-measurement and epistemic narrowing. This makes it more urgent than ever to return to a plural vision of value, capable of guiding the digital transformation in ways that are not only efficient but also just, inclusive, and humane.

Financing Healthcare: From Fee-for-Service to Value-Based Models

This section examines how payment models both reflect and shape changing notions of value in healthcare, highlighting their role in the broader transformation of clinical priorities, organizational structures, and social contracts.

The Limits of Fee-for-Service and the Emergence of Prospective Payment

The concept of "value" in healthcare has not only transformed clinical paradigms and organizational logics but has also exerted a profound influence on the methods by which healthcare systems are financed. Funding mechanisms are not devoid of bias; rather, they embody specific visions concerning what constitutes quality care, the appropriate providers of such care, and the equitable distribution of resources.

Over time, as healthcare systems have reoriented their focus—from volume to quality, from individual interventions to coordinated care, and from provider-centric models to approaches centered on patients and populations—so too have the financing models evolved, adapting to these emerging normative and operational priorities.

Historically, numerous healthcare systems, particularly in high-income nations, have been constructed upon fee-for-service (FFS) paradigms. Within this framework, healthcare providers receive reimbursement for each individual service, procedure, or consultation delivered. The FFS system corresponds with the prestational care model, whereby activity volume is equated with productivity and value. This system was originally designed to reward clinical efforts and to ensure accessibility to care; however, over time, it became apparent that FFS engendered strong incentives for overprovision, fragmentation, and rising costs. Healthcare providers exhibited minimal motivation to coordinate care, eliminate duplication, or prevent hospital admissions. Furthermore, FFS did not adequately account for the quality or outcomes of the services provided.

The United States exemplifies a paradigmatic case of fee-for-service (FFS) dominance, particularly within its private insurance-driven sector. For decades, the majority of healthcare providers received reimbursement on a per-procedure or per-visit basis, thereby fostering a system in which high-technology, specialist-led care was prioritized over preventative or primary care. As healthcare expenditures escalated—surpassing 17% of gross domestic product (GDP) by the early 2020s—criticism intensified regarding the inefficiency and inequity inherent in this model. Consequently, policymakers initiated experiments with alternative payment models (APMs), including bundled payments, capitation, and shared savings programs (e.g., Medicare's Accountable Care Organizations). These models aimed to realign financial incentives with value-based principles, incentivizing providers based on outcomes, cost containment, and patient satisfaction, rather than the volume of care delivered.

Simultaneously, European welfare states, despite their structural differences from the United States, experienced substantial transformations. In nations such as France, Germany, Italy, and the Nordic countries, healthcare is predominantly publicly funded, universal, and founded on the principles of solidarity. However, many of these systems initially implemented prestitial payment schemes, particularly in hospital care. Public hospitals were frequently reimbursed on a per-day or per-procedure basis, reflecting—albeit within a public framework—the same inefficiencies observed in private systems.

Beginning in the 1980s and 1990s, numerous European nations embarked on a transition toward prospective payment frameworks, most prominently through the implementation of diagnosis-related groups (DRGs). Within DRG structures, hospitals are compensated with a predetermined sum for the treatment of patients categorized under specific diagnostic groups, independent of the actual resources consumed. This represented a pivotal shift: rather than rewarding service volume, DRGs promote efficiency. Hospitals are now financially driven to abbreviate hospital stays, diminish superfluous interventions, and adopt more proactive cost management strategies.

For example, in Italy, the national adoption of DRGs in the mid-1990s was part of a broader effort to contain public expenditure and introduce managerial logics into the National Health Service. Similarly, in Germany, the 2003 reform introduced DRGs to increase transparency, foster competition among hospitals, and reduce variation in costs. In France, the *Tarification à l'activité (T2A)* followed a comparable rationale. These changes reflected a shift from the centrality of the medical act to the performance of the healthcare institution, reconfiguring hospitals as semi-autonomous actors responsible for balancing clinical outcomes with economic stewardship.

Value-Based Payment: Promise and Pitfalls

However, while DRGs improved cost control and made hospital performance more measurable, they also introduced new tensions. Critics noted that DRGs could promote "gaming" behaviors, such as upcoding (classifying cases in higher-paying categories) or premature discharges. Moreover, because DRGs are largely focused on acute care, they are ill-suited to addressing chronic conditions, multimorbidity, or long-term care—areas increasingly central in aging societies. Additionally, DRGs risked penalizing hospitals serving disadvantaged populations, whose patients often require more complex and longer treatments.

The progression of funding models has advanced through the proliferation of value-based payment (VBP) methodologies, which are inspired by the conceptual framework of value-based healthcare (VBHC). These models endeavor to establish a direct correlation between financing and quantifiable outcomes, such as hospital readmission rates, infection rates, or patient-reported outcome measures (PROMs). In the United Kingdom, for instance, the National Health Service (NHS) has incorporated elements of VBP through initiatives such as the Best Practice Tariff and the Commissioning for Quality and Innovation (CQUIN). Similarly, the Dutch healthcare system, characterized by a regulated competition model, has conducted trials with bundled payments and integrated care contracts designed to incentivize coordination and preventive measures. In the United States, analogous trends are evident in programs such as Medicare's quality payment program and the implementation of accountable care organizations, which seek to realign financial incentives toward value rather than volume.

Nevertheless, just as the VBHC model has been critiqued for its economic reductionism, VBP mechanisms face similar criticisms. By focusing narrowly on specific indicators, these models risk neglecting contextual and relational aspects of care and may create perverse incentives to focus on what is measurable rather than what is meaningful. Moreover, outcome-based payments require robust data infrastructures, reliable risk-adjustment methodologies, and shared definitions of quality—conditions not always present, especially in less digitized systems.

Hybrid and Equity-Oriented Models for a Digital Era

Today, we find ourselves at a pivotal crossroads. The digital transformation of healthcare, coupled with increasing demands for sustainability, equity, and accountability, necessitates the development of innovative financing models. These models must transcend the traditional dichotomy of FFS versus DRG or activity-based versus outcome-based approaches. Instead, they should encapsulate the intricate nature of healthcare as a relational, social, and systemic enterprise.

Emerging approaches point toward hybrid models, which blend population-based funding (e.g., for primary care networks), capitation, and performance incentives, tailored to local contexts. There is also growing interest in financing models that reward equity, continuity of care, and social value—elements typically absent from traditional funding schemes.

This evolution emphasizes the intricate relationship between healthcare financing reforms and broader social and economic frameworks. In European welfare states, reforms commonly align with principles of solidarity and universal access, thereby reflecting societal commitments to equity and social protection. Conversely, in the United States, reforms tend to prioritize market efficiency, individual responsibility, and competition, embodying the economic and cultural values inherent in its healthcare system. Both contexts demonstrate that financial models function not merely as technical mechanisms but also as representations of societal priorities, thereby shaping and being shaped by the social contract among citizens, healthcare providers, and the State.

The European Commission, in its 2019 report *"Defining Value in 'Value-Based Healthcare'"*, underlines that sustainability in healthcare financing must be interpreted broadly: not just as cost-effectiveness, but as the ability to ensure long-term access, equity, and trust. Similarly, American policy discussions increasingly recognize the need to balance cost containment with quality and access, amid ongoing debates about healthcare's role in social welfare and economic productivity. In this perspective, the future of healthcare financing will depend not only on metrics and algorithms, but on collective choices about what kind of care we value, for whom, and under which conditions.

Mapping the Risks of Digital Medicine: A Necessary Step Toward Sustainable Transformation

In the preceding chapter, the emphasis was on the barriers to the implementation and adoption of digital medicine—namely, structural, organizational, technical, and cultural obstacles that may impede or complicate its integration into healthcare systems. These encompass limited infrastructure, lack of interoperability, professional resistance, insufficient funding, and regulatory uncertainty. Although barriers hinder the complete realization of digital medicine's potential, they are distinct from risks. Barriers can be mitigated through investment and policy reform; conversely, risks relate to adverse outcomes that may occur even when digital medicine is successfully deployed.

Acknowledging and analyzing risks does not imply a pessimistic stance. On the contrary, it reflects a precautionary, forward-looking, and responsible approach. In a context where digital technologies are increasingly shaping health policies, practices, and everyday life, mapping risks is essential to ensure that transformation is not only efficient and innovative but also fair, ethical, and socially sustainable. The goal is not to halt progress, but to guide it wisely—ensuring that no one is left behind, that new vulnerabilities are not created, and that technological development aligns with shared values and rights.

This section outlines five major domains of risk in digital medicine: social inequalities and exclusion, algorithmic bias and systemic reproduction, medicalization and behavioral pressure, reductionism and epistemic impoverishment, and the shift from patient-centered to system-centered value.

The Risk of New Inequalities and Social Exclusion

Arguably, the most pressing and conspicuous concern pertains to the digital divide, which transcends mere access to devices or internet connectivity. In Europe, approximately 32% of adults lack fundamental digital skills, and only 26% demonstrate above-basic digital competence, with pronounced disparities between urban and rural areas—33% in urban settings compared to 20% in rural regions. In the United States, comparable disparities in digital literacy persist, particularly among older adults, lower-income populations, and non-English speakers. Globally, an estimated 5.64 billion individuals (constituting 68.7% of the world population) are connected to the internet; however, 2.6 billion remain offline, predominantly residing in lower-income and rural areas, thereby accentuating global inequalities. The dissemination of technology is occurring at an unprecedented pace: mobile phones took approximately twenty years to achieve 50% global adoption, social media platforms required only 5–7 years, and ChatGPT reached one million users in merely 5 days. Such rapid acceleration indicates that while digital services are expanding expeditiously, the development of digital skills and infrastructure frequently fails to keep pace—thus exacerbating rather than mitigating the digital divide.

In health systems that are progressively integrated with continuous digital connectivity—where appointments, prescriptions, monitoring, and consultations are dependent on digital platforms—individuals lacking requisite skills or reliable connectivity are at heightened risk of social exclusion. Older adults, persons with disabilities, socioeconomically disadvantaged groups, linguistic minorities, and individuals with limited educational backgrounds encounter compounded digital barriers. Substandard connectivity—characterized by unstable mobile networks, limited data access, and sluggish broadband—further impairs usability and access, especially within rural or marginalized communities.

These are not just technical issues—they are deeply social. Health systems that overlook them may inadvertently reinforce existing disparities. For example, digital triage tools prioritizing self-reporting and rapid input can misclassify patients with language, cognitive, or digital barriers, leaving them underserved. Dependency on app-based follow-up can also erode provider–patient relationships, especially for those needing human assistance to navigate health pathways.

It is therefore essential that equity impact assessments be embedded within the planning and evaluation of digital health programs. Solutions must be designed and tested with diverse populations, not only the digitally fluent. Otherwise, rapid digital rollouts risk reinforcing both national and global digital divides—leveraging speed without anchoring in inclusion.

Uneven Digital Literacy Among Healthcare Professionals: The Risk of a Two-Tier Health System

Closely associated with the overarching issue of the digital divide is the unequal distribution of digital skills among healthcare professionals, which raises concerns regarding the development of a dual-tiered healthcare system. Although digital transformation endeavors to enhance care coordination, efficiency, and access, its effectiveness is largely dependent on the preparedness, training, and confidence of the workforce. When this readiness is inconsistent, entire institutions or regions may consequently be at a disadvantage.

Healthcare professionals practicing in remote, underserved, or structurally disadvantaged regions may face significant challenges in accessing ongoing education programs, peer support, or current technological advancements. In these settings, clinicians are often anticipated to utilize sophisticated digital tools—such as telemedicine platforms, electronic health records, clinical decision support systems, or AI-enabled diagnostics—despite insufficient training, limited time, or inadequate infrastructure. This situation results in inconsistent adoption, fragmented utilization, and occasionally, active resistance.

The consequences are not solely operational but also systemic in nature. Facilities lacking digitally proficient personnel may be regarded as less advanced or secure, thereby perpetuating existing disparities in healthcare delivery and reputation. Patients residing in such areas may be deprived of innovations accessible elsewhere, resulting in what may be characterized as "digital deserts" within national health systems. The potential exists for the inadvertent creation of a landscape composed of "A-class" and "B-class" hospitals, distinguished not solely by geographic location or funding but also by levels of digital maturity.

Furthermore, compelling untrained professionals to utilize unfamiliar technologies may lead to heightened stress levels, diminished job satisfaction, and sensations of inadequacy or burnout. These emotional and professional pressures can intensify the pre-existing shortages of healthcare workers in regions that are challenging to staff, thereby further enlarging the disparity between high-resource and low-resource settings.

Addressing this risk necessitates a comprehensive commitment to inclusive digital capacity development, involving targeted investments in education, mentorship, infrastructure, and support mechanisms. Training should be regarded not as an ancillary component but as an integral part of digital implementation strategies. Specifically, it is essential to adopt a context-sensitive approach, acknowledging the distinct needs of various healthcare settings and eschewing uniform digital deployment strategies.

Ultimately, digital transformation will only be as equitable as the systems that support it. Equipping healthcare professionals with the essential skills and confidence is not merely a technical matter; it is a strategic imperative for the development of just, efficient, and resilient health systems in the digital era.

Algorithmic Bias and the Reproduction of Systemic Imbalances

Digital medicine relies significantly on diverse data sources—structured and unstructured, clinical and behavioral, real-time and historical. Algorithms developed from these datasets are employed to assess risk, allocate resources, propose diagnoses, and enhance treatment strategies. However, data are not inherently neutral; they are social constructs influenced by the systems responsible for their collection and by the historical biases ingrained within these systems.

Numerous studies have demonstrated that health algorithms can perpetuate and even amplify inequalities. For instance, risk prediction models may underdiagnose conditions in women or people of color if the training datasets are skewed toward white male populations. Insurance scoring systems might penalize individuals living in deprived areas due to proxies like zip codes or employment status. Even hospital admission algorithms have been shown to allocate fewer resources to Black patients compared to white patients with similar clinical needs.

These algorithmic distortions do not arise from malicious intent, but from implicit biases in data collection, variable selection, and model design. Once implemented at scale, however, they can systematically disadvantage certain groups, leading to inequitable care pathways, resource misallocation, and erosion of trust.

To mitigate this, transparency, accountability, and participation are crucial. Patients and communities must have the right to understand how algorithms affect their care, and there must be clear processes for auditing and contesting algorithmic decisions. Moreover, developers must be encouraged—and mandated where appropriate—to test for and correct bias, and to design with inclusion in mind from the outset.

The Medicalization of Everyday Life and the Pressure to Perform Health

Digital medicine is progressively integrating into everyday life through wearables, fitness trackers, remote monitoring devices, and health-related smartphone applications. Although these tools provide significant benefits for preventive care and the management of chronic diseases, they also pose the risk of obscuring the distinction between medical necessity and lifestyle enhancement, thus promoting a paradigm of perpetual surveillance and self-monitoring.

In this paradigm, health is no longer regarded as a collective right or a shared responsibility, but instead is considered a moral obligation and an individual duty. Individuals are expected to monitor their steps, manage their glucose levels, measure their heart rate variability, and modify their behaviors accordingly—often under the scrutiny of employers, insurers, or digital platforms. The pervasive pressure to engage in perpetual self-improvement may induce anxiety, guilt, and self-blame, particularly among those who find it challenging to meet normative health benchmarks.

This shift contributes to what some scholars refer to as the "quantified self" society, wherein individual value is progressively linked to quantifiable biological parameters. Additionally, it mirrors a broader trend toward the commodification of health—where wellness is transformed into a marketplace, and health data assumes the role of currency.

There is an increasing necessity to scrutinize the psychosocial consequences of this model. Are we fostering a culture in which solely the "optimally healthy" are regarded as responsible citizens? Are we endangering a form of health elitism, wherein the capacity to handle data and optimize performance constitutes a new axis of inequality? A more sustainable approach would acknowledge the relational, emotional, and environmental facets of health—dimensions that are not readily captured by sensors and dashboards.

The Reduction of Health to What Is Measurable

One of the most subtle yet far-reaching risks in digital medicine is the epistemic narrowing of what is considered valuable knowledge. Digital systems prioritize what can be quantified, coded, and standardized—yet healthcare remains deeply contextual, narrative, and relational.

As digital tools become central in evaluating clinical performance, planning services, and allocating resources, there is a tendency to favor what is measurable over what is meaningful. This may result in an undervaluation of nonquantifiable aspects, such as listening, trust, empathy, cultural understanding, or community integration. Moreover, the prioritization of quantifiable outcomes may skew care delivery toward biomedical metrics, neglecting psychosocial needs and social determinants of health. In primary care, for example, clinicians may be pushed to prioritizing the achievement of digital targets (such as screening rates and medication adherence) over engaging in extensive, complex dialogues that genuinely address patients' lived experiences represents a concerning trend. This "quantitative drift" also bears significant implications for the training and professional identity of future clinicians. There is a risk that upcoming healthcare professionals may be socialized into a care model that equates quality solely with metrics, rather than with ethical commitments or relational presence. Such a tendency not only threatens dehumanization but also leads to epistemic impoverishment—a constriction of what is regarded as valid knowledge within the medical field. To mitigate this, it is essential to advocate for multiple epistemologies. This encompasses qualitative insights, experiential knowledge, community voices, and cultural narratives. Technological innovations should aim to enhance, rather than supplant, these vital dimensions of care.

The Risk of Algorithmic Drift: From Value for the Patient to Value for the System

Finally, a critical risk lies in the conceptual drift that occurs when the ideal of "value for the patient" is gradually supplanted by value for the system. In value-based digital health frameworks, efficiency, cost-effectiveness, and performance indicators can become dominant metrics—sometimes at the expense of patient agency, professional autonomy, or ethical nuance.

This drift is especially evident in automated decision-making, where clinical pathways are optimized for throughput or cost savings rather than individualized care. It also appears in policy frameworks that reward system-level efficiencies without adequately accounting for patient experience or cultural appropriateness.

While system sustainability is a legitimate concern—especially in aging societies with constrained budgets—there is a danger that systemic rationality overrides ethical deliberation. A digital triage tool that excludes patients with "low expected benefit" may be economically sound, but ethically fraught. A hospital that reduces readmissions through aggressive discharge planning may improve its performance score, but harm vulnerable patients.

To prevent this, value must be contextualized, plural, and relational. Sustainability in healthcare must be understood not only in terms of financial efficiency but also through a broader lens that includes social equity, ethical responsibility, and long-term human impact. A truly sustainable system is one that balances economic viability with fairness, inclusiveness, and the capacity to respond to the diverse needs of individuals and communities. Digital medicine should strive to balance efficiency with equity, proximity, participation, and respect for diversity.

In conclusion, digital medicine holds extraordinary promise. But as with all powerful tools, it brings with it the possibility of unintended consequences. Recognizing risks is not a sign of distrust or resistance—it is a condition of mature, inclusive, and sustainable innovation.

Planning for the future of healthcare must go beyond technical feasibility and economic efficiency. It must ask: Whose interests are served? Whose voices are heard? What kinds of futures are we building? By systematically mapping risks, we create the possibility of doing better—not only technologically, but socially and ethically.

Addressing Risks and Shaping the Future of Digital Medicine: Toward Inclusive and Equitable Innovation

Recognizing the risks associated with digital medicine is not a call to slow progress—it is a necessary step to shape it wisely. The potential of digital technologies to improve healthcare systems, empower patients, and support professionals is enormous. However, to fully realize this potential, we must actively work to map, anticipate, and mitigate the systemic risks they bring. This requires a strategic, coordinated, and values-driven approach—one that balances technological innovation with social sustainability, and efficiency with justice.

A fundamental initial step involves the incorporation of equity frameworks into the conception and assessment of digital health initiatives. Frequently, digital health solutions are created in isolated silos—technologically proficient yet socially insensitive. Principles of equity-by-design must be implemented from the beginning, guaranteeing that systems are not only user-friendly but also inclusive, adaptable, and sensitive to context. This process encompasses comprehensive impact assessments, collaborative design with diverse user groups, and continuous monitoring of disparities in access, utilization, and outcomes.

In parallel, investing in digital health literacy at all levels is essential. This entails not only providing training for patients and citizens but also for clinicians, administrators, and policymakers. The capacity to understand, evaluate, and effectively utilize digital tools should be regarded as a fundamental competence in contemporary healthcare—rather than a discretionary skill. Customized, accessible, and ongoing training programs are required, especially in underserved regions and for professionals with limited digital proficiency. Furthermore, initiatives should incorporate considerations for the emotional and relational aspects of learning, offering support systems that acknowledge apprehension, resistance, and fatigue.

Equally important is the need to protect the relational and ethical core of healthcare. Digital medicine must not reduce care to measurable outputs or automated interactions. Instead, it should be designed to enhance human connections, free time for relationships, and support trust and empathy. This includes resisting the "quantification trap," where only what can be measured is valued, and acknowledging the epistemic richness of clinical intuition, dialogue, and contextual judgment. Digital tools should support—not replace—these human dimensions.

Regarding governance, it is imperative to prioritize comprehensive frameworks for responsible data utilization and algorithmic transparency. Patients and healthcare professionals should have the right to comprehend, scrutinize, and regulate the collection, processing, and application of health data. This encompasses ensuring the explainability of algorithms, safeguarding against biases and misuse, and facilitating meaningful consent procedures.

Data governance must also be founded on the principle of collective responsibility, harmonizing individual rights with public health imperatives and involving diverse stakeholders in decision-making processes. Another key avenue lies in rethinking how we define and measure value in healthcare. As discussed earlier, narrow conceptions of value—focused solely on economic efficiency or technical outcomes—fail to capture what matters most to people. A pluralistic vision of value must guide digital innovation, one that includes dignity, proximity, participation, continuity, and cultural appropriateness. In this light, models such as the "triple value" framework—combining personal, allocative, and technical value—offer a more holistic orientation. However, even these models must be adapted to the complexity of real-world contexts, recognizing the diversity of health needs, expectations, and social determinants.

To implement these principles effectively, it is essential to institutionalize patient and community engagement throughout the entire lifecycle of digital initiatives. This entails surpassing mere surveys or pilot tests and fostering co-creation practices whereby end-users play an active role in defining the objectives, features, and evaluation standards of digital tools. Instruments such as PROMs (patient-reported outcome measures) and PREMs (patient-reported experience measures) can act as conduits toward a more democratic healthcare system, provided they are integrated within authentic participatory processes.

Looking ahead, the future of digital medicine will depend not only on technological breakthroughs but also on our collective ability to govern innovation in a socially just manner. This includes resisting the temptation to over-centralize or commodify care, and instead promoting models of distributed, context-sensitive, and culturally competent innovation. It means supporting local capacities, reducing dependency on large digital monopolies, and fostering open-source, interoperable systems that serve the public good.

International cooperation will also be essential. Supranational institutions possess a pivotal role in establishing ethical standards, harmonizing regulations, and fostering cross-border collaboration. Shared principles of equity, transparency, and sustainability should underpin national and regional strategies, ensuring that digital transformation benefits health as a universal public good.

In conclusion, it is imperative to recognize that time stands as one of the most valuable resources within the realm of care. Digital medicine ought not to hasten systems to the point of exhaustion, but rather to liberate time for activities such as listening, understanding, and providing support. This necessitates a paradigm shift in innovation: embracing depth as well as speed, fostering relationships alongside automation, and prioritizing efficiency in conjunction with the quality of care. Irrespective of the social values inherent in a given system, proactively identifying and evaluating risks enhances collective awareness and mitigates unforeseen disruptions, thereby promoting a more resilient and adaptable digital transformation.

Case Studies and Exercises: Applying a Critical Lens to Digital Value

To consolidate the insights discussed in this chapter and translate them into actionable understanding, this final section offers real-world case studies and hands-on exercises. These are designed to stimulate critical thinking, foster interdisciplinary dialogue, and support professionals in applying a values-based, inclusive approach to digital transformation in healthcare.

Case Studies

Case Study #1—Algorithmic Bias in Risk Prediction Tools
Context: A US hospital system uses an AI-based triage algorithm to prioritize patients for chronic disease management programs. An external audit reveals that Black patients, despite similar clinical profiles, are assigned lower risk scores than white patients.

Discussion Focus: Identify where bias may have entered the system. What corrective actions (data enrichment, model retraining, participatory auditing) could have been taken earlier?

Case Study #2—DRGs and Early Discharge Pressures
Context: An Italian hospital operating under the DRG payment system begins discharging elderly patients with multimorbidity prematurely to avoid financial losses. Readmissions rise sharply.

Discussion Focus: Explore the tension between economic efficiency and clinical appropriateness. How could a hybrid model better address complexity and care continuity?

Case Study #3—Digital Deserts in Rural Healthcare
Context: A telemedicine initiative is launched across a European region, but uptake in rural areas remains low due to poor connectivity and limited digital literacy among healthcare workers.

Discussion Focus: Design an equity-by-design response strategy. What forms of support, investment, and training are needed to close this gap?

Case Study #4—Quantification vs. Relational Care
Context: A Scandinavian primary care clinic implements a KPI-driven quality dashboard. Over time, doctors report decreased morale and less time for nonmeasurable care (e.g., palliative conversations, social concerns).

Discussion Focus: How can performance evaluation systems integrate qualitative dimensions? What is lost when empathy and presence are not captured by metrics?

Case Study #5—Patient Participation in Digital Tool Development
Context: A health authority develops a remote monitoring app for post-surgery care without involving patients in the design phase. Usage is low, and many find the interface unintuitive or alienating.

Discussion Focus: Redesign the development process using co-creation principles. How could PROMs and PREMs be used not only for evaluation but for iterative design?

Practical Exercises

Exercise #1—Mapping Value Perspectives
Using the Triple Value Model (Personal, Allocative, Technical), select a digital health tool (e.g., glucose monitor, teleconsultation platform). Identify how each type of value is addressed—or overlooked—in its current use.

Exercise #2—Risk Assessment Grid
Develop a structured risk matrix for a new AI diagnostic tool. Include categories such as digital exclusion, algorithmic bias, overmedicalization, and loss of relational care. Propose mitigation strategies for each.

Exercise #3—Narrating the "Quantified Self"
Write a fictional narrative or diary entry from the perspective of a patient under constant self-monitoring (e.g., wearable fitness and sleep tracker). Reflect on the psychological and social implications of continuous surveillance.

Exercise #4—Policy Brief Simulation
Draft a one-page policy brief for your country's health ministry advocating for equity-by-design principles in national digital health initiatives. Include rationale, examples, and key actions.

Exercise #5—Audit Your System
Select a local or institutional digital health service (e.g., online booking, e-prescription). Assess it through an inclusion and ethics lens: Who may be excluded? What biases might be present? What changes could make it more just?

Final Thoughts: Charting a Human-Centered Path for Digital Medicine

As digital medicine continues to expand its reach across health systems worldwide, it is vital to remember that technology is never neutral—it reflects the values, priorities, and power structures of the societies in which it is embedded. This chapter has highlighted how the promise of digital transformation must be weighed against the risk of deepening inequality, narrowing our epistemic horizons, and inadvertently shifting the focus of care from the person to the system. The challenge is not whether we should embrace digital tools—this transformation is already underway—but how we do so, and on whose terms. A conscious, ethically grounded, and socially inclusive approach is not a luxury—it is a necessity. Innovation must not only be faster or smarter, but also more equitable, more participatory, and more attuned to the lived realities of diverse individuals and communities. If value in healthcare is to mean more than efficiency or profitability, then the digital future must be governed with plural values at its core: care, dignity, solidarity, and trust. The digital age offers a unique opportunity—not only to reform healthcare systems—but to reimagine them as more just, compassionate, and human.

Suggested Reading

1. Porter ME. What is value in health care? N Engl J Med. 2010;363(26):2477–81. https://doi.org/10.1056/NEJMp1011024.
2. Porter ME, Teisberg EO. Redefining health care: creating value-based competition on results. Boston: Harvard Business School Press; 2006.
3. Boltanski L, Thévenot L. On justification: economies of worth. Princeton, NJ: Princeton University Press; 2006 [orig. 1991].
4. Marx K. Capital: a critique of political economy, vol. 1. Hamburg: Meissner; 1867.
5. Weber M. Economy and society: an outline of interpretive sociology. Berkeley, CA: University of California Press; 1978 [orig. 1922].
6. European Commission. Defining value in "value-based healthcare": report of the expert panel on effective ways of investing in health (EXPH). Brussels: European Commission; 2019.
7. Boltanski L, Thévenot L. Orders of worth: on justification in economics, politics and law. Brazillier; [French orig. 1991].
8. Gentili A, Failla G, Melnyk A, et al. The cost-effectiveness of digital health interventions: a systematic review of the literature. Front Public Health. 2022;10:787135. https://doi.org/10.3389/fpubh.2022.787135.
9. Eurostat. Digital skills and competence statistics – Statistics Explained. 2021. Available at: https://ec.europa.eu/eurostat/statistics-explained/index.php?title=Digital_skills_statistics
10. Pew Research Center. Digital divide persists even as lower-income Americans make gains in tech adoption. 2021. Available at: https://www.pewresearch.org/internet/2021/06/22/digital-divide-persists-even-as-lower-income-americans-make-gains-in-tech-adoption/; https://doi.org/10.2139/ssrn.3880384.
11. DataReportal. Digital Around the World 2025. 2025. Available at: https://datareportal.com/reports/digital-2025-global-overview-report
12. International Telecommunication Union (ITU). Measuring digital development: facts and figures 2024. Geneva: ITU Publications; 2024. Available at: https://www.itu.int/en/ITU-D/Statistics/Documents/facts/FactsFigures2024.pdf. https://doi.org/10.18356/5c8508f9-en.
13. Statista. Average adoption rates of new technologies worldwide 2023. Available at: https://www.statista.com/statistics/269025/number-of-social-media-users-worldwide/
14. World Health Organization. WHO guideline: recommendations on digital interventions for health system strengthening. Geneva: WHO; 2019.
15. World Health Organization. Global strategy on digital health 2020–2025. Geneva: WHO; 2021.
16. Teisberg E, Wallace S, O'Hara S. Defining and implementing value-based health care: a strategic framework. Acad Med. 2020;95(5):682–5. https://doi.org/10.1097/ACM.0000000000003122.
17. World Economic Forum. Value in healthcare: laying the foundation for health system transformation. Geneva: World Economic Forum. (Policy report); 2017.
18. World Health Organization. WHO guideline: recommendations on digital interventions for health system strengthening. Geneva: WHO. (Guideline report); 2019.
19. World Health Organization. Global strategy on digital health 2020–2025. Geneva: WHO. (Strategy publication); 2021.
20. World Health Organization. Ethics and governance of artificial intelligence for health: WHO guidance. Geneva: WHO. (Guidance report); 2021.
21. European Commission. Communication on enabling the digital transformation of health and care in the digital single market; empowering citizens and building a healthier society (COM(2018) 233 final). Brussels: European Commission. (Policy communication); 2018.

22. Organisation for Economic Co-operation and Development (OECD). Health in the 21st century: putting data to work for stronger health systems. OECD Health Policy Studies. Paris: OECD Publishing; 2019. https://doi.org/10.1787/e3b23f8e-en.
23. World Bank. Digital-in-health: unlocking the value for everyone. Washington, DC: World Bank. (Policy report); 2023.
24. Obermeyer Z, Powers B, Vogeli C, Mullainathan S. Dissecting racial bias in an algorithm used to manage the health of populations. Science. 2019;366(6464):447–53. https://doi.org/10.1126/science.aax2342.
25. Vyas DA, Eisenstein LG, Jones DS. Hidden in plain sight — reconsidering the use of race correction in clinical algorithms. N Engl J Med. 2020;383(9):874–82. https://doi.org/10.1056/NEJMms2004740.
26. Parikh RB, Teeple S, Navathe AS. Addressing bias in artificial intelligence in health care. JAMA. 2019;322(24):2377–8. https://doi.org/10.1001/jama.2019.18058.
27. Cirillo D, Catuara-Solarz S, Morey C, et al. Sex and gender differences and biases in artificial intelligence for biomedicine and healthcare. Npj Digital Med. 2020;3(1):Article 81. https://doi.org/10.1038/s41746-020-0288-5.
28. Topol EJ. High-performance medicine: the convergence of human and artificial intelligence. Nat Med. 2019a;25(1):44–56. https://doi.org/10.1038/s41591-018-0300-7.
29. Adams J. Ethical and epistemic implications of artificial intelligence in medicine: a stakeholder-based assessment. AI & Society. (Published online 25 May 2025). 2025. https://doi.org/10.1007/s00146-025-02398-4.
30. Ramsetty A, Adams C. Impact of the digital divide in the age of COVID-19. J Am Med Inform Assoc. 2020;27(7):1147–8. https://doi.org/10.1093/jamia/ocaa078.
31. Western MJ, Smit ES, Gültzow T, et al. Bridging the digital health divide: a narrative review of the causes, implications, and solutions for digital health inequalities. Health Psychol Behav Med. 2025;13(1) (in press) https://doi.org/10.1080/21642850.2025.2493139.
32. Topol EJ. Deep medicine: how artificial intelligence can make healthcare human again. New York, NY: Basic Books. (Book); 2019b.
33. Wachter RM. The digital doctor: Hope, hype, and harm at the Dawn of medicine's computer age. New York, NY: McGraw-Hill Education. (Book); 2015.
34. Voorheis P, Petch J, Pham Q, Kuluski K. Maximizing the value of patient and public involvement in the digital health co-design process: a qualitative descriptive study with design leaders and patient-public partners. PLOS Digital Health. 2023;2(10):e0000213. https://doi.org/10.1371/journal.pdig.0000213.
35. Douglas AO, Senkaiahliyan S, Bulstra CA, Mital C, Atun R. Global adoption of value-based health care initiatives within health systems: a scoping review. JAMA Health Forum. 2025;6(5):e250746. https://doi.org/10.1001/jamahealthforum.2025.0746.
36. International Telecommunication Union (ITU). Measuring digital development: facts and figures 2023. Geneva: ITU; 2023. (Public data report)
37. Veinot TC, Mitchell H, Ancker JS. Good intentions are not enough: how informatics interventions can worsen inequality. J Am Med Inform Assoc. 2018;25(8):1080–8. https://doi.org/10.1093/jamia/ocy052.

The Future of Digital Medicine 7

Emerging Technologies to Watch

As Digital Medicine continues to evolve, the pace of technological innovation shows no signs of slowing down. Emerging tools and platforms are enhancing current healthcare capabilities and redefining what is possible across the entire care continuum from prevention and diagnosis to treatment and long-term management. The technologies explored in this section are at the forefront of this transformation, enabling new ways to deliver care, engage patients, and improve outcomes.

Artificial intelligence and machine learning have progressed considerably beyond their initial applications, now encompassing multi-modal data analysis and developing solutions that integrate imaging, genomics, wearable data, and environmental factors into actionable insights. These advancements exemplify a broader trend, initially discussed in Chap. 4, whereby AI-driven tools transform diagnostics and clinical decision-making through the provision of nuanced, patient-specific information. The evolution of explainable AI further enhances this progression by addressing concerns related to transparency and trust, while ensuring that clinicians and patients understand the rationale behind AI recommendations.

Simultaneously, immersive technologies such as augmented reality (AR) and virtual reality (VR) are transforming the education of healthcare providers and the interactions of patients with their health. These tools, which integrate visual and sensory feedback, offer innovative approaches to medical training and more personalized and accessible patient engagement, connecting back to the themes of Chap. 3 regarding how technology humanizes care.

Bioelectronic medicine and implantable devices constitute a significant advancement, integrating hardware and software to attain enhanced compatibility with the human body. Ranging from neural interfaces that interpret brain activity to intelligent textiles that gather real-time health information, these innovations broaden the scope of technological capabilities. They exemplify the principles of personalized

A. Cesario et al., *Digital Medicine Starter Guide*,
https://doi.org/10.1007/978-3-032-01272-2_7

care as outlined in Chap. 2, where technology is customized to address the distinctive needs and conditions of individuals.

Collectively, these technologies demonstrate the significant potential of Digital Medicine to transform healthcare in unprecedented ways, previously considered unimaginable a decade ago. Nonetheless, the effective integration of these innovations requires more than technological expertise; as outlined in Chap. 3, ethical principles, privacy concerns, and regulatory guidelines will be essential to ensure their responsible deployment. The subsequent sections will provide a comprehensive analysis of these emerging technologies, emphasizing their capabilities, challenges, and future implications for healthcare.

The Role of Big Data and Predictive Analytics

The foundation of contemporary Digital Medicine is data—extensive, intricate datasets obtained from numerous sources such as electronic health records (EHRs), wearable devices, genomic sequencing, environmental monitoring systems, and social media activities. These datasets are not merely static archives; rather, they are dynamic resources that, when analyzed judiciously, can reveal extraordinary insights into patient health, healthcare system efficiency, and public health developments. The advancement of big data and predictive analytics is revolutionizing healthcare, facilitating a transition from reactive treatments to proactive and preventive care. Whereas traditional healthcare primarily addressed illnesses post-onset, these innovative tools now enable practitioners to anticipate and avert health crises prior to their manifestation.

The transformative power of big data lies not only in its scale but also in its ability to connect disparate data sources. Combining genomic data with environmental factors, socioeconomic conditions, and patient behavior provides a holistic view of previously unattainable health. As discussed in Chap. 4, this comprehensive integration enhances both individual and population health outcomes, offering clinicians and public health officials the ability to make decisions based on real-time, actionable insights.

Proactive, Population-Level Insights

One of the most significant impacts of big data is its capacity to generate insights across entire populations, thereby informing public health strategies. Predictive analytics, which employs historical and real-time data to forecast future trends, has become an indispensable tool in managing public health crises. For instance, during the COVID-19 pandemic, predictive models played a crucial role in identifying infection hotspots, allocating vital resources such as ventilators and vaccines, and prioritizing interventions for vulnerable populations. These applications, as detailed in Chap. 4, demonstrate how big data enables healthcare systems to respond effectively to large-scale challenges.

Beyond emergency situations, predictive analytics facilitates risk stratification, thereby enabling healthcare systems to categorize populations based on their risk profiles for chronic diseases, including diabetes, asthma, and cardiovascular disorders. Through the analysis of neighbourhood-level data, health authorities can pinpoint regions with high prevalence rates and implement targeted interventions, such as mobile clinics, community health programs, and specialized telehealth services. This emphasis on equity is consistent with the themes presented in Chap. 1, which underscored the significance of ensuring access to care for underserved populations.

Moreover, the advancement of large-scale data analytics is propelling the development of precision public health, which focuses on customizing interventions for individuals as opposed to demographic groups. Through the integration of genomic data with lifestyle, environmental, and behavioral factors, public health initiatives are capable of providing highly targeted solutions that optimize effectiveness while reducing inefficiencies. For instance, in the realm of precision oncology, predictive models can ascertain which patients are likely to gain the most benefit from particular screening programs or genetic testing, thereby enabling earlier diagnosis and improving health outcomes.

Personalized Care Pathways

While Big Data offers insights at the population level, its most substantial impact may be found in the transformation of individual care. Real-time analytics empower clinicians to devise personalized care pathways that adapt dynamically to a patient's evolving needs. For instance, predictive models and biomarkers in oncology are increasingly utilized to monitor patient responses to treatments, enabling clinicians to adjust therapies in real time. This concept of adaptive treatment, discussed in Chap. 2, minimizes the trial-and-error approach that has traditionally characterized cancer care, thereby reducing costs and enhancing patient experiences.

Wearable devices and mobile health applications have also emerged as essential enablers of personalized healthcare. By continuously monitoring metrics such as heart rate variability, glucose levels, and physical activity, these tools empower patients to assume greater control over their health. For instance, devices such as Abbott's FreeStyle Libre provide individuals with diabetes ongoing glucose monitoring, thereby enabling them to promptly adjust their diet, exercise regimen, or medication. These tools, examined in Chap. 3, serve to bridge the gap between patients and healthcare providers, fostering a more collaborative and participatory model of care.

Predictive analytics enhances personalization and transforms healthcare into an anticipatory system. By identifying early warning signs of disease, clinicians can intervene prior to the exacerbation of symptoms or the emergence of complications. For instance, remote monitoring systems that track vital signs in patients with heart failure can notify providers of subtle changes, thereby facilitating timely adjustments to treatment plans. This proactive approach, closely aligned with the 4P healthcare model (predictive, preventive, personalized, and participatory), signifies a fundamental shift in health management.

The New Frontiers of Integrated Care

Healthcare fragmentation has long been a barrier to optimal outcomes. Siloed systems, where providers, specialities, and care settings operate independently, lead to inefficiencies, redundant tests, and inconsistent communication. Emerging integrated care models aim to address these challenges by creating seamless, connected systems that prioritize the patient experience and deliver coordinated care across the continuum.

Hospital-at-Home/Virtual Hospital Models

The hospital-at-home model represents one of the most innovative approaches to integrated care. This model enables patients to receive high-quality care for acute and post-acute conditions without leaving their homes by leveraging advances in telemedicine, remote monitoring devices, and portable diagnostic tools. This approach has proven particularly beneficial for patients with chronic illnesses, post-surgical recovery needs, or conditions requiring intensive monitoring but not hospitalization.

Programs such as the Mount Sinai Hospital at Home initiative have demonstrated considerable advantages, including reduced costs, a lower incidence of hospital-acquired infections, and elevated patient satisfaction rates. For instance, patients recovering from pneumonia may be equipped with wearable devices designed to monitor vital signs, including oxygen saturation and heart rate, while engaging in daily virtual check-ins with their healthcare team. Portable diagnostic tools, such as handheld ultrasound devices, can be utilized as necessary, ensuring that patients receive comprehensive care without the physical or emotional burdens associated with a hospital stay.

This model underscores the significance of multidisciplinary collaboration. Pharmacists, nurses, and therapists collaborate with physicians to deliver comprehensive care, ensuring that all facets of patient recovery are duly considered. As referenced in Chap. 5, these coordinated initiatives augment accessibility and mitigate disparities, especially for patients in rural or underserved regions.

All-in-One Digital Health Platforms

With the increasing adoption of digital tools, a new challenge has emerged: fragmentation within the realm of Digital Medicine. Patients and healthcare providers frequently experience difficulty due to the necessity of navigating multiple platforms and applications, each tailored to a specific function, such as telehealth consultations, wearable data analysis, or medication management. Comprehensive Digital Health platforms endeavor to address this concern by integrating these disparate functionalities into a unified interface.

Platforms such as Epic's MyChart and Cerner's HealtheLife exemplify this trend by unifying electronic health record (EHR) data, wearable metrics, telemedicine services, and appointment scheduling into a comprehensive overview of a patient's health. This integration not only streamlines workflows for healthcare professionals but also enhances the patient experience, thereby reducing the complexity associated with managing their care.

These platforms also facilitate continuous care teams, wherein multidisciplinary providers can access shared data streams to coordinate interventions with seamless efficiency. For instance, a cardiologist, a nutritionist, and a primary care physician can collaborate on a patient's care plan, ensuring that each decision is informed by a comprehensive understanding of the patient's needs. This reflects the team-based approach discussed in Chap. 2, where patient-centered care models were demonstrated to enhance outcomes and satisfaction.

As digital health platforms gain sophistication, it is anticipated that they will integrate predictive analytics and artificial intelligence-driven insights, thereby empowering healthcare providers to foresee patient needs and enhance the delivery of care. This evolution is in harmony with the overarching objectives of digital medicine: to develop a healthcare system that is not only efficient but also profoundly personalized and participatory.

Adaptive Legislation

As Digital Medicine becomes an integral component of healthcare systems globally, regulatory frameworks must adapt to effectively address the distinct challenges and opportunities it presents. One of the most significant developments in this domain is the European Health Data Space (EHDS), an initiative led by the European Union aimed at facilitating the secure and standardized sharing of health data among member states. In conjunction with the Data Governance Act (DGA), which offers broader guidance on data sharing and governance across various sectors, the EHDS serves as a fundamental pillar in Europe's endeavors to spearhead the global health data revolution.

The EHDS aims to achieve two key objectives:

1. *Empower citizens by granting them comprehensive control over their health data and ensuring.*
2. *They have ready access to it, irrespective of their location within the European Union.*

and facilitate the secondary utilization of health data for research, innovation, and public health purposes while maintaining stringent privacy and security standards.

Under the framework of the European Health Data Space (EHDS), patients are granted the opportunity to access their medical records electronically, thereby facilitating seamless continuity of care while traveling or seeking treatment in another European Union (EU) member state. For example, a patient visiting a medical facility in Spain can provide a physician with real-time access to their medical history from their country of origin. This level of integration considerably mitigates the redundancy of tests and examinations, reduces costs, and enhances the overall quality of care. Chapter 3, which addresses interoperability challenges, underscores the vital role of such initiatives in establishing a cohesive healthcare ecosystem.

The Data Governance Act (DGA) complements the European Health Data Space (EHDS) by providing a legal foundation for the sharing of data across various sectors, ensuring that sensitive information, including health data, is managed in an ethical and secure manner. It introduces mechanisms such as "data altruism," wherein individuals voluntarily share their anonymized health data for the public good, particularly for purposes such as medical research or public health initiatives. These frameworks are designed to enhance innovation and cultivate public trust—a theme that is explored in Chap. 7, where privacy and transparency are discussed as essential components for fostering patient confidence in digital tools.

Together, the EHDS and the Data Governance Act establish a foundation for a future in which health data is regarded as both a personal asset and a collective resource aimed at improving healthcare outcomes across Europe. Furthermore, these initiatives serve as a model for other regions striving to balance innovation with ethical data management.

Patient Empowerment and the Shift to Wellness

The healthcare paradigm is undergoing a significant transformation. Previously, the primary emphasis was placed on the treatment of illness; however, healthcare systems are now evolving to prioritize wellness, prevention, and patient empowerment. The capacity of Digital Medicine to engage patients as active participants in their healthcare is driving this change. It utilizes technology to enhance the accessibility, personalization, and proactivity of health management.

From Episodic to Continuous Care

Historically, healthcare interactions have been episodic in nature. Patients typically consult a healthcare provider solely when symptoms manifest, frequently after the progression of a medical condition. Digital Medicine is transforming this paradigm by facilitating continuous care, in which wearable devices, home diagnostic tools, and interconnected platforms deliver real-time insights into patient health.

For instance, individuals managing chronic conditions such as diabetes or hypertension are no longer required to wait for a quarterly check-up to evaluate their health status. Devices such as continuous glucose monitors (CGMs) and blood pressure cuffs that connect to mobile applications enable daily monitoring, generating valuable data that patients and healthcare providers can utilize to dynamically adjust treatment plans. This evolution reflects the themes discussed in Chap. 2, where it was demonstrated that patient-generated health data significantly enhances health outcomes.

Continuous care also facilitates early intervention. Predictive algorithms, driven by real-time data, can notify healthcare providers of subtle alterations in a patient's health prior to their manifestation as acute symptoms. This proactive strategy diminishes hospitalizations, reduces healthcare expenses, and enhances quality of life.

Informed Decision-Making

A principal obstacle to patient empowerment has historically been the intricacy of medical information. Numerous patients encounter challenges in understanding medical terminology, treatment alternatives, and the implications of their choices. Digital tools are effectively bridging this gap by converting complex data into practical insights.

For instance, artificial intelligence-driven virtual assistants and chatbots can provide patients with personalized explanations concerning their medical conditions, prescribed medications, and treatment protocols. Platforms such as Ada Health and Babylon Health utilize conversational AI to guide patients through their symptoms, deliver preliminary assessments, and suggest subsequent steps. As elaborated in Chap. 4, these tools not only enhance health literacy but also render healthcare more accessible to individuals who may find traditional clinical environments intimidating.

In addition to digital assistants, data visualization dashboards fundamentally alter the engagement with health data. By illustrating metrics such as blood pressure trends and glucose levels in an intuitive visual format, these dashboards empower patients to monitor their progress, set objectives, and participate collaboratively in decision-making with healthcare providers. As emphasized in Chap. 3, shared decision-making fosters collaboration, thereby ensuring that patients feel recognized and respected throughout their care journey.

Wellness as a Priority

Digital Medicine is also redirecting its focus from "sick care" to authentic preventive Wellness. Rather than addressing health issues solely after their onset, technology empowers individuals to sustain Wellness through lifestyle modifications and early interventions.

Wearable devices, such as the Apple Watch and Fitbit, are at the forefront of preventive health, continuously monitoring key metrics including heart rate variability, sleep patterns, and activity levels. When complemented by AI-driven insights, these devices are capable of providing personalized recommendations, such as promoting increased physical activity, suggesting stress-reduction techniques, or notifying users of potential health risks. Furthermore, at the community level, wellness programs may aggregate data obtained from these devices to discern trends and devise targeted interventions, a concept closely aligned with the discussion in Chap. 1 regarding equitable access to digital tools.

Nutrition, mental health, and environmental factors are integral components of wellness strategies. Digital health platforms now furnish customized meal plans predicated on genetic profiles, mindfulness applications deliver personalized stress management programs, and environmental sensors monitor air quality to inform individuals regarding potential respiratory risks. By addressing these encompassing determinants of health, digital medicine transcends traditional clinical care to adopt a holistic perspective on well-being.

The Role of Gamification and Community

Numerous digital platforms are integrating gamification and community support to enhance patient engagement in their wellness journeys. Applications such as Noom and MyFitnessPal employ goal-setting, rewards, and social sharing to promote adherence to health and wellness initiatives. These strategies are particularly effective in facilitating long-term behavioral change, as they leverage intrinsic motivations and cultivate a sense of accountability.

Furthermore, online health communities furnish patients with a platform to share their experiences, seek guidance, and extend support. These communities, frequently hosted on Digital Health platforms, cultivate a sense of belonging and alleviate the isolation experienced by numerous patients. Additionally, they function as invaluable resources for the exchange of practical tips and strategies for managing chronic conditions.

Case Studies and Practical Exercises

Case Studies

Case Study #1: Google DeepMind's AlphaFold in Precision Medicine

Summary: AlphaFold, an artificial intelligence system created by DeepMind, has profoundly transformed the realm of protein structure prediction, yielding substantial progress in drug discovery and precision medicine. Through the integration of artificial intelligence with genomic and proteomic data, researchers are able to identify novel disease pathways and accelerate the formulation of targeted therapies.

Key Takeaways: Explore how AI is revolutionizing drug discovery, the thrilling integration of multimodal data, and what these advancements signify for personalized medicine.

Case Study #2: Stanford Medicine's Use of VR for Surgical Training

Summary: Stanford Medicine has successfully integrated virtual reality into its surgical training programs, allowing medical students to practice complex procedures within a virtual environment. This immersive technology has significantly improved procedural accuracy and reduced errors in practical applications.

Key Takeaways: Enhanced medical training, reduction of skill gaps, improving patient outcomes through AR/VR.

Case Study #3: Neuralink's Brain–Computer Interface (BCI)

Summary: Neuralink, an enterprise established by Elon Musk, is engaged in the development of brain–computer interfaces (BCIs) that facilitate direct communication between the human brain and digital devices. These implants possess the potential to restore mobility in individuals affected by paralysis and to revolutionize the field of neurorehabilitation.

Key Takeaways: Future of brain-machine interfaces, ethical concerns, potential applications in neurotherapy.

Case Study #4: AI-Driven Pandemic Response—BlueDot

Summary: BlueDot, an artificial intelligence-based public health surveillance organization, detected the COVID-19 outbreak several days prior to the World Health Organization's initial warnings by analyzing global travel patterns and epidemiological data. This predictive methodology facilitated early intervention and enhanced preparedness.

Key Takeaways: Predictive analytics in epidemiology, early warning systems, public health preparedness.

Case Study #5: IBM Watson and AI-Driven Oncology Care

Summary: IBM Watson has been employed in oncology to analyze extensive datasets and propose personalized cancer treatment plans. Through the integration of genomic, clinical, and real-world patient data, artificial intelligence enhances precision medicine and improves treatment efficacy.

Key Takeaways: AI in oncology, personalized treatment pathways, improving patient outcomes.

Case Study #6: Mount Sinai's Hospital-at-Home Program

Summary: The Mount Sinai Health System has instituted a hospital-at-home program, facilitating eligible patients to access acute care in the comfort of their residences through the utilization of telemedicine, remote monitoring, and in-home nursing assistance. This initiative has resulted in decreased costs, diminished occurrences of hospital-acquired infections, and enhanced patient satisfaction.

Key Takeaways: Cost-effective acute care, benefits of home-based monitoring, improved patient experience.

Case Study #7: Epic's MyChart—Unified Patient Engagement

Summary: Epic's MyChart integrates patient health records, wearable data, telehealth services, and medication management into a unified platform. This integration enhances patient engagement, streamlines care coordination, and delivers real-time health insights.

Key Takeaways: Benefits of Digital Health consolidation, interoperability challenges, enhanced patient autonomy.

Case Study #8: European Health Data Space (EHDS) Initiative

Summary: The European Union's Electronic Health Data Space (EHDS) seeks to establish standardized protocols for sharing health data among its member states, while ensuring rigorous privacy protections. This initiative not only facilitates cross-border healthcare services but also enhances research capabilities and improves patient access to their personal health data.

Key Takeaways: Standardizing Digital Health governance, privacy considerations, and cross-border data interoperability.

Case Study #9: Algorithmic Bias in AI—The COMPAS Controversy

Summary: The COMPAS AI system, employed within the United States criminal justice framework, revealed instances of racial bias in its risk assessment methodologies. This case highlights the imperative for transparency and equity in healthcare AI models to avert biased medical decision-making.

Key Takeaways: Ethical AI governance, transparency in machine learning, addressing bias in Digital Medicine.

Case Study #10: Abbott's FreeStyle Libre for Diabetes Management

Summary: Abbott's FreeStyle Libre provides continuous glucose monitoring, which enables individuals with diabetes to make real-time adjustments to their lifestyle and medication. This technology has profoundly improved glycemic control and patient outcomes autonomy.

Key Takeaways: Benefits of real-time monitoring, patient engagement, impact on chronic disease management.

Case Study #11: Ada Health—AI-Powered Patient Education

Summary: The AI chatbot developed by Ada Health assists users in conducting symptom assessments and provides personalized health information, thereby enhancing health literacy and facilitating patient care decision-making.

Key Takeaways: AI for patient empowerment, improving health literacy, reducing unnecessary clinical visits.

Practical Exercises

Exercise #1: Evaluating an Emerging Digital Health Technology

Task: Select an emerging technology (e.g., AI-driven diagnostics, VR-based therapy, neural interfaces) and evaluate its potential impact on patient care, regulatory considerations, and ethical concerns.

Reflection Question: In what ways can healthcare providers ensure the responsible and equitable implementation of this technology?

Exercise #2: Designing a Predictive Analytics Framework for Public Health

Task: Assume the role of a developer creating a public health surveillance system utilizing predictive analytics; identify key data sources (e.g., EHRs, wearable data, social determinants of health) and define key performance indicators (KPIs) to measure success.

Reflection Question: How can predictive analytics be employed to enhance interventions in population health?

Exercise #3: Developing a Hospital-at-Home Model

Task: Design a hospital-at-home model tailored for a specific condition (e.g., post-surgical recovery, heart failure management); outline the necessary digital tools, remote monitoring capabilities, and strategies for provider-patient engagement.

Reflection Question: What obstacles must be addressed to successfully scale hospital-at-home programs?

Exercise #4: Creating a Regulatory Roadmap for Digital Medicine

Task: Choose a Digital Health innovation (e.g., AI diagnostics, blockchain for health records) and identify the relevant regulatory frameworks (e.g., GDPR, HIPAA, FDA); propose a compliance strategy that ensures patient safety and data privacy.
Reflection Question: How can adaptive regulations evolve to keep pace with rapidly advancing Digital Health innovations?

Exercise #5: Enhancing Patient Engagement Through Gamification

Task: Design a Digital Health application that integrates gamification to improve patient adherence; outline reward mechanisms, community features, and functionalities for behavior tracking.
Reflection Question: In what ways does gamification affect long-term patient engagement and health outcomes?

Final Thoughts

This chapter offers a forward-thinking yet structured approach to emerging Digital Medicine trends by incorporating case studies and practical exercises. These components provide readers with real-world insights into how AI, big data, immersive technologies, and predictive analytics will influence the future of healthcare while tackling ethical, regulatory, and patient empowerment challenges.

Suggested Reading

1. Topol EJ. High-performance medicine: the convergence of human and artificial intelligence. Nat Med. 2019;25(1):44–56.
2. Yu KH, Beam AL, Kohane IS. Artificial intelligence in healthcare. Nat Biomed Eng. 2018;2(10):719–31.
3. Kelly CJ, Karthikesalingam A, Suleyman M, Corrado G, King D. Key challenges for delivering clinical impact with artificial intelligence. BMC Med. 2019;17(1):195.
4. Baker A, Perov Y, Middleton K, Baxter J, Mullarkey D, Sangar D, et al. A comparison of artificial intelligence and human doctors for the purpose of triage and diagnosis. Front Artif Intell. 2020;3:543405.
5. Obermeyer Z, Powers B, Vogeli C, Mullainathan S. Dissecting racial bias in an algorithm used to manage the health of populations. Science. 2019;366(6464):447–53.
6. Vayena E, Haeusermann T, Adjekum A, Blasimme A. Digital health: meeting the ethical and policy challenges. Swiss Med Weekly. 2018;148:w14571.

7. High-Level Expert Group on Artificial Intelligence (European Commission). Ethics guidelines for trustworthy AI. Brussels: European Commission; 2019.
8. World Health Organization. Ethics and governance of artificial intelligence for health. Geneva: WHO; 2021.
9. World Health Organization. WHO guideline: recommendations on digital interventions for health system strengthening. Geneva: WHO; 2019.
10. World Health Organization. Global strategy on digital health 2020–2025. Geneva: WHO; 2021.
11. Dorsey ER, Topol EJ. Telemedicine 2020 and the next decade. The Lancet. 2020;395(10227):859.
12. Mandel JC, Kreda DA, Mandl KD, Kohane IS, Ramoni RB. SMART on FHIR: a standards-based, interoperable apps platform for electronic health records. J Am Med Informatics Assoc. 2016;23(5):899–908.
13. Holmgren AJ, Patel V, Adler-Milstein J. Progress in interoperability: measuring US hospitals' engagement in sharing patient data. Health Affairs. 2017;36(10):1820–7.
14. JASON (The MITRE Corporation). A robust health data infrastructure. Agency for Healthcare Research and Quality; 2014. AHRQ Publication No. 14-0041-EF
15. Matheny ME, Thadaney-Israni S, Ahmed M, Whicher D, editors. Artificial intelligence in health care: the hope, the hype, the promise, the peril. Washington, DC: National Academy of Medicine; 2019.
16. Silcox C, Zimlichman E, Huber K, Rowen N, Saunders R, McClellan M, Bates DW. The potential for artificial intelligence to transform healthcare: perspectives from international health leaders. NPJ Digit Med. 2024;7:88. https://doi.org/10.1038/s41746-024-01097-6.
17. Topol EJ. High-performance medicine: the convergence of human and artificial intelligence. Nat Med. 2019;25(1):44–56. https://doi.org/10.1038/s41591-018-0300-7.
18. Kickbusch I, Piselli D, Agrawal A, Balicer R, Banner O, Xue L. The Lancet and Financial Times Commission on governing health futures 2030: growing up in a digital world. The Lancet. 2021;398(10312):1727–76. https://doi.org/10.1016/S0140-6736(21)01824-9.
19. World Health Organization. Ethics and governance of artificial intelligence for health: WHO guidance. Geneva: World Health Organization; 2021. https://www.who.int/publications/i/item/9789240029200
20. World Health Organization. Global strategy on digital health 2020–2025. Geneva: World Health Organization; 2021. https://www.who.int/docs/default-source/documents/gs4dh-daa2a9f352b0445bafbc79ca799dce4d.pdf
21. Ratti E, Morrison M, Jakab I. Ethical and social considerations of applying artificial intelligence in healthcare – a two-pronged scoping review. BMC Med Ethics. 2025;26:68. https://doi.org/10.1186/s12910-025-01198-1.
22. Vorisek CN, Lehne M, Klopfenstein SAI, Mayer PJ, Bartschke A, Haese T, Thun S. Fast Healthcare Interoperability Resources (FHIR) for interoperability in health research: systematic review. JMIR Med Informatics. 2022;10(7):e35724. https://doi.org/10.2196/35724.
23. Cripps M, Scarbrough H. Making digital health "solutions" sustainable in healthcare systems: a practitioner perspective. Front Digit Health. 2022;4:727421. https://doi.org/10.3389/fdgth.2022.727421.
24. Organisation for Economic Co-operation and Development. Health in the 21st century: putting data to work for stronger health systems. Paris: OECD Publishing; 2019. https://www.oecd.org/en/publications/health-in-the-21st-century_e3b23f8e-en.html
25. Meskó B, Kristóf T, Dhunnoo P, Árvai N, Katonai G. Exploring the need for medical futures studies: insights from a scoping review of health care foresight. J Med Internet Res. 2024;26:e57148. https://doi.org/10.2196/57148.
26. Katsoulakis E, Wang Q, Wu H, Shahriyari L, Fletcher R, Deng J. Digital twins for health: a scoping review. NPJ Digit Med. 2024;7:77. https://doi.org/10.1038/s41746-024-01073-0.
27. European Medicines Agency. Reflection paper on the use of artificial intelligence in the medicinal product lifecycle. Amsterdam: EMA; 2024. https://www.ema.europa.eu/en/documents/scientific-guideline/reflection-paper-use-artificial-intelligence-ai-medicinal-product-lifecycle_en.pdf

28. Carrero ZI, Eckardt JN, Ghaffari Laleh N, Löffler CML, Schwarzkopf S-C, Kather JN. The future landscape of large language models in medicine. Commun Med. 2023;3:141. https://doi.org/10.1038/s43856-023-00370-1.
29. Wilhelm TI, Kaczmarczyk R, Al-Dulaimi R, Eltorai AEM, Agrawal S, Flahault A. Decoding the digital pulse: bibliometric analysis of 25 years in digital health research through the Journal of Medical Internet Research. J Med Internet Res. 2024;26(1):e60057. https://doi.org/10.2196/60057.
30. World Health Organization. WHO guideline: recommendations on digital interventions for health system strengthening. Geneva: World Health Organization; 2019. https://www.who.int/publications/i/item/9789241550505
31. Food US, Administration D. Artificial Intelligence/Machine Learning (AI/ML)-based software as a medical device action plan. Silver Spring: FDA; 2021.
32. Organisation for Economic Co-operation and Development. Health data governance for the digital age: implementing the OECD recommendation on health data governance. Paris: OECD Publishing; 2022. https://www.oecd.org/en/publications/health-data-governance-for-the-digital-age_68b60796-en.html
33. Kaboré SS, Ngangue P, Soubeiga D, Barro A, Pilabré AH, Savadogo GBL. Barriers and facilitators for the sustainability of digital health interventions in low- and middle-income countries: a systematic review. Front Digit Health. 2022;4:1014375. https://doi.org/10.3389/fdgth.2022.1014375.
34. Ewoh P, Vartiainen T. Vulnerability to cyberattacks and sociotechnical solutions for health care systems: systematic review. J Med Internet Res. 2024;26(1):e46904. https://doi.org/10.2196/46904.
35. Topol E. The Topol review: preparing the healthcare workforce to deliver the digital future. London: NHS Health Education England; 2019. https://topol.hee.nhs.uk/the-topol-review/
36. Mandl KD, Kohane IS. A 21st-century health IT system – creating a real-world information economy. New Engl J Med. 2017;376(20):1905–7. https://doi.org/10.1056/NEJMp1700235.
37. Organisation for Economic Co-operation and Development. The COVID-19 pandemic and the future of telemedicine. Paris: OECD Publishing; 2023. OECD Health Working Papers No. 142
38. Babu M, Lautman Z, Lin X, Sobota MHB, Snyder MP. Wearable devices: implications for precision medicine and the future of health care. Annu Rev Med. 2024;75:401–15. https://doi.org/10.1146/annurev-med-052422-020437.
39. Rajkomar A, Dean J, Kohane IS. Machine learning in medicine. N Engl J Med. 2019;380(14):1347–58. https://doi.org/10.1056/NEJMra1814259.
40. European Commission High-Level Expert Group on AI. Ethics guidelines for trustworthy AI. Brussels: European Commission; 2019. https://digital-strategy.ec.europa.eu/en/library/ethics-guidelines-trustworthy-ai

Conclusion: The New Era of Digital Medicine

8

Digital Medicine: A Transformation in Motion

Digital Medicine transcends mere fleeting trends or a mere assemblage of disruptive technologies; it epitomizes the evolution of healthcare into a fully interconnected, data-driven, and patient-centered system. This transformation is propelled by the convergence of emerging tools, ethical imperatives and an urgent necessity to confront the challenges faced by traditional healthcare systems in the present day. However, as this book has elucidated, the journey is anything but linear. The transition requires a delicate equilibrium of innovation, regulation, and trust.

This volume has intricately woven a narrative of Digital Medicine that transcends isolated technologies to address its systemic impact on the essence of care delivery. Each chapter aspires to connect the dots between conceptual principles, real-world applications, and forward-looking visions, while never losing sight of the ultimate objective: a more equitable, accessible, and effective healthcare system.

A Cohesive Vision: Revisiting Key Themes

The narrative commenced with Chap. 1, establishing the foundation by identifying the essential pillars of Digital Medicine: predictive, preventive, personalized, and participatory care (4P healthcare). These principles are not abstract ideals; they signify the fundamental shift necessary to reimagine care. For example, the transition from episodic interactions to continuous engagement—facilitated by wearable devices, real-time monitoring, and mobile health platforms—embodies this transformation.

Chapters 2 and 3 subsequently investigated the tools that actualize this vision, ranging from telemedicine and AI-driven diagnostics to mHealth applications and biosensors. These instruments constitute the scaffolding of Digital Medicine, presenting the potential to not only enhance care delivery but also democratize access

A. Cesario et al., *Digital Medicine Starter Guide*,
https://doi.org/10.1007/978-3-032-01272-2_8

to it. The principles of interoperability and clinical validation, introduced early in the book, resonate throughout these chapters, highlighting the necessity for technologies that integrate seamlessly into clinical workflows while upholding the highest standards of safety and efficacy.

The intricacies of implementation took center stage in Chaps. 4 and 5, where we delved into the significant barriers to adoption—cultural, financial, regulatory, and infrastructural. These chapters reminded us that technological innovation, irrespective of its sophistication, cannot thrive in isolation. It must be complemented by thoughtful strategies that address tangible constraints, whether through phased implementation, fostering digital literacy, or cultivating trust through transparency and ethical governance.

Chapter 6 expanded the narrative by shifting the focus from technological capabilities to the broader societal implications of Digital Medicine. Drawing from sociological theory, this chapter unpacked the evolving definitions of "value" in healthcare—from clinical outcomes and economic efficiency to symbolic and relational dimensions of care. It examined how digital tools, when framed exclusively through technocratic lenses or narrow performance metrics, risk entrenching inequities, eroding trust, and alienating vulnerable populations. Yet, the chapter also illuminated a path forward: a vision of Digital Medicine that is not only intelligent and efficient but also conscious and just. Through this lens, innovation becomes meaningful only when it aligns with ethical imperatives, embraces complexity, and remains anchored in the lived realities of diverse patient communities.

The narrative culminated in Chap. 7, which envisioned a future shaped by emergent technologies such as bioelectronic medicine, big data analytics, and immersive platforms like augmented reality. These innovations present breathtaking possibilities—from transforming diagnostics to redefining patient engagement. Yet, as underscored throughout this book, their deployment must adhere to the principles of equity and sustainability. The technologies of tomorrow will only realize their full potential if they cater to the broadest possible audience, transcending barriers of geography, socioeconomic status, and digital literacy.

Bridging Innovation and Humanity

As we conclude this exploration, one truth emerges clearly: Digital Medicine is not solely about technology—it is fundamentally about humanity. It entails harnessing data and tools to address disparities, empower patients, and deliver care that embodies empathy alongside efficiency. However, this requires more than mere technological progress. It necessitates a cultural shift, wherein healthcare providers, patients, policymakers, and innovators collaborate to construct a system that aligns with shared values.

Trust serves as the cornerstone of this vision. Patients must trust that their data remains secure, clinicians must have confidence in the tools they employ, and communities must believe that these advancements will benefit the greater good. Throughout this volume, the interplay between trust, innovation, and equity has emerged as a recurring theme, underscoring the delicate balance essential to ensure that the digital revolution leaves no one behind.

A Call to Action

The future of Digital Medicine lies within our collective ability to shape it. As policymakers formulate adaptive regulations, clinicians adopt new workflows, technologists refine their tools, and patients become more actively engaged in their care, the possibilities are boundless. Nonetheless, this transformation will only succeed if we confront the systemic barriers, ethical dilemmas, and inequities that impede progress.

The journey ahead is as complex as it is promising. Nevertheless, by aligning innovation with purpose and progress with empathy, we can construct a healthcare system that embodies the best of what Digital Medicine presents—one that is not only technologically advanced but is also profoundly human at its core.

Appendices

Appendix A: Future Technologies Relevant to Digital Medicine

Agentic Artificial Intelligence

Agentic artificial intelligence (AI) signifies a transformative advancement in the evolution of intelligent systems. While traditional AI systems perform tasks within narrowly defined boundaries, agentic AI introduces the capability to self-initiate actions, pursue goals, and make context-sensitive decisions with a greater degree of autonomy. This emerging category of AI builds upon reinforcement learning, large language models, and multi-agent systems, often designed to perceive environments, adaptively respond to stimuli, and operate across complex tasks without continuous human supervision.

In the context of digital medicine, agentic AI has the potential to revolutionize patient care and health system operations. Intelligent agents could, for instance, monitor patient data in real time, autonomously trigger clinical alerts, personalize treatment pathways, and coordinate with other digital health tools across varying care settings. Agentic systems may also optimize hospital logistics, predict equipment failures, or even manage health interventions at the population level, particularly during outbreaks or chronic disease surveillance. A compelling example is the deployment of AI-powered care navigators, which guide patients through complex treatment pathways by leveraging both structured and unstructured health data.

However, agentic AI also presents significant challenges. Its ability for autonomous decision-making raises questions about clinical accountability, transparency, and trust. The "black-box" nature of advanced AI systems often complicates explainability—a crucial factor in healthcare. Ethical dilemmas regarding autonomy, bias propagation, consent, and the delegation of decision-making to machines require thorough discussion and careful regulatory frameworks. The emergence of agentic AI calls for strong governance structures to ensure these technologies align with patient safety, medical ethics, and societal values.

Looking ahead, research in agentic AI is advancing rapidly, with interdisciplinary initiatives integrating behavioural science, neuroscience, robotics, and biomedical informatics. As these systems evolve, the healthcare sector must prepare to

A. Cesario et al., *Digital Medicine Starter Guide*,
https://doi.org/10.1007/978-3-032-01272-2

engage with them not just as tools, but as partners in care delivery. The future of agentic AI in digital medicine relies on balancing its powerful capabilities with human oversight, ethical integrity, and public trust.

Blockchain in Digital Medicine

Blockchain technology, originally developed to support decentralized financial systems, is making significant strides in the digital health sector as a robust infrastructure for trust, transparency, and secure data exchange. At its core, blockchain is a distributed ledger technology that records transactions in a tamper-proof, cryptographically linked chain, ensuring integrity and verifiability without relying on centralized authorities.

In healthcare, blockchain offers numerous use cases with direct implications for digital medicine. Among the most promising is the secure management of electronic health records (EHRs), enabling interoperable and patient-controlled data exchange across institutions. Blockchain can also be used to ensure the integrity of clinical trial data, allowing regulators and researchers to verify time-stamped entries and audit trails in real time. Another application lies in supply chain management for pharmaceuticals and medical devices, where blockchain ensures traceability, authenticity, and quality assurance throughout the lifecycle of critical assets.

From a privacy and interoperability standpoint, blockchain provides significant advantages. Smart contracts—self-executing code embedded in the blockchain—can automate consent management, ensuring that data sharing respects patient preferences and regulatory requirements. Moreover, the decentralized architecture minimizes the risk of single points of failure and makes large-scale data breaches harder to achieve. When combined with federated learning and edge computing, blockchain-based systems could facilitate AI training on distributed datasets without compromising privacy.

Nevertheless, several barriers hinder mainstream adoption. Scalability remains a core concern, as most public blockchain systems struggle with transaction throughput and latency. Energy efficiency, especially in proof-of-work models, presents environmental and operational challenges. Additionally, regulatory uncertainty and the lack of unified standards complicate integration with existing healthcare infrastructure. The necessary cultural shift—from institution-centered to trustless, distributed ecosystems—also requires change management and stakeholder engagement.

Despite these challenges, pilot projects and research consortia are paving the way for blockchain-enabled digital health ecosystems. Governments and academic institutions are exploring hybrid models that combine the immutability of blockchain with compliance-focused architectures. The trajectory suggests that blockchain, while not a cure-all, will play a foundational role in developing secure, interoperable, and patient-centered digital medicine infrastructures.

Quantum Computing in Digital Medicine

Quantum computing is set to redefine computational paradigms by harnessing the principles of quantum mechanics—superposition, entanglement, and quantum tunneling—to conduct complex calculations at unprecedented speeds. While it is still in the early stages of maturity, the implications for healthcare and digital medicine are extensive.

One of the most anticipated applications of quantum computing is in drug discovery and molecular modeling. Classical computers struggle to simulate the behavior of large biomolecules due to the exponential complexity of quantum interactions. In contrast, quantum computers can natively process quantum states, which allows the simulation of protein folding, molecular docking, and receptor binding with a level of accuracy that could drastically accelerate the development of new therapies. This capability has the potential to significantly shorten discovery timelines and reduce costs.

In the field of bioinformatics and genomics, quantum algorithms have the potential to improve pattern recognition and dimensionality reduction for large-scale omics data. Machine learning models driven by quantum computing might eventually enable highly personalized medicine by integrating multi-modal datasets—genetic, environmental, and behavioral—into predictive health models. Furthermore, quantum-enhanced optimization could be utilized for designing clinical trials, allocating healthcare resources, or simulating the spread of infectious diseases.

However, the transition from theoretical promise to real-world application is constrained by technological and infrastructural limitations. Quantum computers are sensitive to environmental noise, require cryogenic conditions, and lack the strong error correction mechanisms necessary for high-fidelity results. Current quantum devices are primarily suited for exploratory research, and their integration into clinical workflows remains uncertain.

Ethical and regulatory considerations must also evolve to address the unique characteristics of quantum computing. Issues regarding algorithmic transparency, data sovereignty, and the implications of quantum-enabled decryption of existing encrypted data must be tackled proactively. The potential for both positive and negative disruptive impacts necessitates global dialogue and anticipatory governance.

In summary, quantum computing represents a frontier technology with transformative potential for digital medicine. Its advancement will require ongoing investment, interdisciplinary collaboration, and regulatory foresight. As it matures, quantum computing may unlock capabilities that redefine how we understand, prevent, and treat diseases in the twenty-first century.

Metaverse and Digital Medicine

The metaverse in digital medicine encompasses immersive virtual environments wherein patients, clinicians, and students can interact in real-time via avatars and extended reality (XR) interfaces. This convergence of physical and digital realms in healthcare is pioneering new frontiers for medical training, patient engagement, and remote care. For instance, surgical trainees and medical students leverage virtual reality simulations and augmented reality guidance to practice intricate procedures in risk-free settings, thereby enhancing their skills and confidence prior to real-life applications. Patients reap the benefits of immersive therapeutic experiences, such as VR-based rehabilitation exercises or virtual support groups, which bolster engagement and adherence by rendering care more interactive and personalized. Furthermore, "virtual hospitals" and telepresence technologies facilitate remote care models in which consultations, monitoring, and even certain treatments can be administered within a shared virtual space, potentially broadening access to specialists irrespective of geographic boundaries. Nonetheless, these opportunities are accompanied by considerable challenges: technical obstacles such as interoperability and substantial hardware costs need to be surmounted for seamless integration into health systems, and ethical considerations assume critical importance. Issues pertaining to data privacy, security, and patient safety are magnified within metaverse platforms, as sensitive health information and realistic avatars circulate in cyberspace. Additionally, there exist concerns regarding equity and access, which necessitate ensuring that all patient populations can benefit from these innovations without exacerbating the digital divide. Nevertheless, the metaverse's potential to revolutionize healthcare is profound. By providing immersive, collaborative, and patient-centric experiences, it has the capacity to enhance medical education outcomes, fortify patient–provider connections, and construct more resilient remote care infrastructures. The realization of this promise will necessitate meticulous governance and ongoing technological refinement, yet the trajectory indicates that virtual environments will increasingly become an integral facet of healthcare delivery and learning in the forthcoming years.

Appendix B. Chapter Snapshots

Chapter 1. Setting the Stage: Understanding Digital Medicine

This chapter highlights the transformative potential of Digital Medicine, focusing on the 4P model: predictive, preventive, personalized, and participatory healthcare. It introduces the societal and technological forces that are propelling this change and discusses the critical themes of accessibility, equity, and sustainability that serve as the foundation of the book.

Chapter 2. The Foundations of Digital Medicine

This chapter examines the fundamental principles that characterize Digital Medicine, emphasizing the pivotal role of data-driven care, ethical considerations, and interoperability. Furthermore, it underscores how evidence-based validation and regulatory frameworks guarantee that digital tools are effective and reliable, thereby establishing a foundation for transformative healthcare innovation.

Chapter 3. Digital Tools and Applications

This chapter investigates the practical applications of Digital Medicine, encompassing telemedicine, mobile health applications, wearables, and AI-driven diagnostics. By demonstrating how these technologies enable continuous care, empower patients, and seamlessly integrate into clinical workflows, it underscores their potential to revolutionize healthcare delivery.

Chapter 4. Implementing Digital Medicine in Clinical Practice

This chapter establishes a connection between theoretical frameworks and practical application, providing a comprehensive roadmap for the effective adoption of digital tools within clinical settings. It evaluates the assessment of organizational needs, the selection of appropriate technologies, integration with established workflows, and the management of prevalent challenges. Furthermore, it explores practical strategies for change management, workforce training, and the measurement of impact.

Chapter 5. Overcoming Barriers to Digital Medicine Adoption

Financial, cultural, and infrastructural obstacles frequently hinder digital transformation. This chapter explores these challenges and presents practical solutions, encompassing innovative reimbursement models, privacy protections, and strategies aimed at bridging the digital divide. It emphasizes the importance of cultivating trust and digital literacy among stakeholders.

Chapter 6. Risks and Opportunities of Digital Medicine

This chapter adopts a sociological perspective to critically examine how digital innovation redefines the concept of value in healthcare. Drawing on classical and contemporary social theory, it explores the tensions between efficiency, equity, and symbolic meaning in the deployment of digital tools such as AI, wearables, and telemedicine. While these technologies promise measurable outcomes and system-level improvements, they may also introduce new forms of exclusion, surveillance, and dehumanization if not carefully governed. The chapter underscores the need for a conscious digital transition—one that harmonizes innovation with ethical responsibility, social justice, and the relational dimension of care.

Chapter 7. The Future of Digital Medicine

Looking ahead, this chapter explores the advanced technologies and care models shaping the future of Digital Medicine. It examines the influence of multimodal artificial intelligence, bioelectronics, big data analytics, and integrated platforms on healthcare innovation. Focus is on empowering patients, evolving regulatory frameworks, and the need for equitable and sustainable healthcare systems.

Appendix C: A Note on the Contextual Major Legislation Relevant to Digital Medicine

As digital medicine advances and integrates more thoroughly into healthcare systems globally, the necessity for a coherent, reliable, and interoperable regulatory framework becomes paramount. Regulatory clarity not only guarantees patient safety and public trust but also lays the groundwork upon which innovation can be responsibly scaled. Although the legislative landscape varies significantly across regions, several major frameworks have emerged as foundational elements of digital medicine governance, establishing standards for data protection, clinical validation, software regulation, and ethical deployment.

Within the European Union, the General Data Protection Regulation (GDPR) stands as a fundamental pillar of privacy legislation. Implemented in 2018, the GDPR governs the methods of collection, processing, and transfer of personal data—including health-related information—while establishing the principle of data minimization and emphasizing user consent, transparency, and the right to erasure. In the domain of digital medicine, which frequently involves real-time health monitoring and cross-border data exchange, adherence to the GDPR is of paramount importance. Closely associated with this is the evolving framework of the European Health Data Space (EHDS), a legislative initiative designed to facilitate the secure and ethical reuse of health data across Europe for purposes such as research, innovation, policy-making, and patient empowerment. The EHDS aims to enhance interoperability between health systems while reinforcing robust data governance mechanisms. In conjunction with these data-centric frameworks, the EU Medical Device Regulation (MDR) oversees the classification, conformity assessment, and post-market surveillance of digital tools, including Software as a Medical Device (SaMD). Under the MDR, developers of digital health applications must demonstrate clinical safety and performance, ensure comprehensive cybersecurity measures, and adhere to harmonized technical standards. The forthcoming AI Act further broadens this regulatory framework by introducing a risk-based approach to the governance of AI systems, encompassing those employed in medical contexts.

In the United States, regulatory oversight is distributed among various agencies, with the Food and Drug Administration (FDA) fulfilling a crucial role. The FDA's Digital Health Innovation Action Plan, along with subsequent guidance documents, establishes a regulatory framework for mobile health applications, clinical decision support tools, and diagnostics based on artificial intelligence. The concept of Software as a Medical Device (SaMD), initially developed in collaboration with the International Medical Device Regulators Forum (IMDRF), has been thoroughly embraced by the FDA, which continuously refines its strategy concerning adaptive algorithms and real-world evidence. Simultaneously, the Health Insurance

Portability and Accountability Act (HIPAA) ensures the protection of personal health information by instituting security and privacy mandates that all digital health systems are required to follow. Although HIPAA was originally designed for conventional healthcare providers, its scope has been expanded through enforcement discretion and interpretive guidance to include emerging digital platforms and remote care modalities. Another significant piece of legislation is the 21st Century Cures Act, which mandates data interoperability and patient access to health information—both of which serve as fundamental enablers of digital medicine. This legislation undergirds the "information blocking" regulations that prevent healthcare entities from hindering the flow of clinical data, thereby enhancing transparency and empowering patients.

Beyond the European Union and the United States, several other jurisdictions have established frameworks that influence the digital medicine landscape. In Canada, the Personal Information Protection and Electronic Documents Act (PIPEDA) regulates the management of personal data by private organizations, including health technology firms, while Health Canada's regulatory pathways for digital health technologies increasingly align with international best practices. In Asia, a variety of national strategies are emerging. Singapore's Personal Data Protection Act (PDPA) is closely aligned with the principles of the General Data Protection Regulation (GDPR) and promotes secure health data initiatives such as the National Electronic Health Record (NEHR). The government of Japan, under its "Society 5.0" vision, has integrated digital health within a broader innovation strategy, emphasizing responsible artificial intelligence, intersectoral collaboration, and data integration. The World Health Organization (WHO) also assumes a significant normative role by issuing global guidelines on digital health interventions that prioritize evidence generation, equity, and governance. These guidelines serve as a reference point for lower- and middle-income countries as they develop regulatory capacity.

Cross-cutting subjects continue to influence the advancement of regulations concerning digital medicine. The ethical implementation of artificial intelligence, particularly within clinical environments, has catalyzed a surge of policy development focused on bias, transparency, and accountability. The European Union's proposed AI Act introduces a multifaceted risk classification system, with medical applications frequently categorized as "high-risk," thereby subjecting them to comprehensive scrutiny. Simultaneously, concerns surrounding cybersecurity have taken on a pivotal role: regulations increasingly necessitate preventative risk assessments, incident response protocols, and the incorporation of security-by-design principles at every stage of digital product development. Challenges related to data sovereignty—particularly when health data is processed through cloud services across diverse jurisdictions—are driving initiatives aimed at localizing infrastructure or establishing cross-border protective measures. Lastly, human rights-based approaches are gaining momentum, with numerous governments and international organizations emphasizing the significance of inclusion, accessibility, and nondiscrimination in digital health.

In conclusion, the regulatory ecosystem governing digital medicine is characterized by its complexity and ongoing evolution, reflecting the multidisciplinary essence of the field. It necessitates the involvement of stakeholders—clinicians, developers, policymakers, and researchers—who must engage not only with local compliance obligations but also with international standards that increasingly influence the parameters of responsible innovation. As digital tools become further integrated into healthcare delivery systems, the capacity to adeptly navigate these frameworks will ultimately dictate both the pace and quality of advancement.

Appendix D: The ABC of the Medical Device Regulation (EU/2016/745)

Risk Classification Criteria for SaMD Under MDR

The EU Medical Device Regulation (MDR) 2017/745 establishes specific rules for classifying Software as a Medical Device (SaMD) based on risk. Notably, Rule 11 of Annex VIII (Classification Rules) addresses stand-alone software:

(a) Software created for the purpose of facilitating diagnostic or therapeutic decisions is categorized as a minimum of Class IIa, unless such decisions could potentially result in death or irreversible health deterioration (in which instance it is classified as Class III), or lead to serious health deterioration or necessitate surgical intervention (whereupon it is designated as Class IIb).
(b) Software designed to monitor physiological processes is classified as Class IIa, except in cases where it is intended to monitor vital physiological parameters that may result in immediate danger to the patient, in which case it is classified as Class IIb.
(c) All other software: Any other standalone software that serves a medical purpose is designated as Class I by default.

Consequently, Rule 11 significantly reclassifies the majority of medical software into higher categories. Almost no standalone medical software remains classified as Class I under the Medical Device Regulation (MDR). Nearly all software intended for diagnosis, prognosis, monitoring, or treatment "provides information to drive decisions," thereby resulting in classification as Class IIa or higher. The practical implication of this regulation is that many Software as a Medical Device (SaMD) that were previously self-certified under the former directives now require oversight from a Notified Body (NB). As noted by the German expert group EK-Med, this rule particularly urges applications to be categorized into higher classes, necessitating the involvement of a Notified Body and potentially requiring clinical trials to ensure compliance.

Manufacturers must meticulously assess the risk class in accordance with Rule 11 to adhere to the appropriate conformity route. It is advisable to consult the MDCG 2019-11 guidance, which aligns Rule 11 with the IMDRF risk framework and provides examples to elucidate borderline cases. In summary, Class I Software as a Medical Device (SaMD) is restricted to those that involve low-risk usage (e.g., solely wellness or preventive functions that do not influence clinical decisions). In contrast, most decision-support or monitoring software will be classified as Class IIa or IIb, while high-criticality algorithms (e.g., those that could potentially cause direct harm to patients if erroneous) may fall into Class III. This classification significantly influences the regulatory pathway, as outlined hereafter.

Step-by-Step Conformity Assessment Process for SaMD (CE Marking)

Acquiring CE marking for Software as a Medical Device necessitates navigating the MDR conformity assessment procedure, which entails fulfilling General Safety and Performance Requirements, assembling comprehensive technical documentation, and typically undergoing a Notified Body review. The principal steps involved are:

Establish a Quality Management System (QMS)

A compliant Quality Management System (QMS) serves as the foundation for conformity with the Medical Device Regulation (MDR). Manufacturers are required to establish a quality system that encompasses design, development, risk management, maintenance, and other aspects pertinent to the device. The majority utilize ISO 13485 as the reference standard. Under the MDR, the implementation of a QMS is obligatory for Class IIa, IIb, and III devices, and it is highly recommended for Class I devices as well. Adhering to ISO 13485 guarantees the documentation of procedures such as design control, verification, software release, post-market surveillance, and others, thereby preparing the organization for the Notified Body's audit. A robust QMS significantly facilitates the compilation and management of the evidence required for the CE marking process.

Develop the Software in Compliance with Key Standards

Throughout the development process, manufacturers are required to adhere to the "state of the art" standards for medical software. The essential standards and normative references include:

(a) ISO 14971 (Risk Management): It is essential to apply a comprehensive risk management process throughout the software lifecycle. This process encompasses the identification of potential hazards (e.g., inaccurate data output, malfunctions, cybersecurity breaches), followed by the estimation and evaluation of associated risks. Appropriate mitigation measures should be implemented, ensuring that any residual risks are deemed acceptable and are outweighed by the derived benefits. Furthermore, it is imperative to maintain a thorough risk management file that links each identified hazard to corresponding controls and the verification of such controls. Compliance with ISO 14971 is explicitly mandated by MDR Annex I.

(b) IEC 62304 (Software Life Cycle Processes): Adhere to a structured software development lifecycle. Categorize the software system's safety class (A, B, or

C) based on risk assessment, and execute processes for planning, requirements management, design, implementation, verification, and maintenance in accordance with IEC 62304. This standard is deemed essential for the CE marking of software, as it provides a framework to substantiate that the software was developed with the requisite rigor. Manufacturers, therefore, ensure that the software "is compliant with all legal requirements, especially IEC 62304 and ISO 14971" to satisfy MDR expectations.

(c) IEC 62366 (Usability Engineering): In instances where the software interface is utilized by patients or clinicians, it is imperative to conduct a usability engineering process to alleviate the potential for use errors. The Medical Device Regulation (MDR) underscores the significance of usability as a component of safety, as stipulated in Annex I, which mandates the reduction of risks stemming from use errors.

(d) Cybersecurity & IEC 81001/MDCG Guidance: Incorporate cybersecurity from design through post-market. MDR Annex I (chapter II) includes requirements for protection against unauthorized access that could create safety risks. Following MDCG 2019-16 guidance on cybersecurity for medical devices (or the newer IEC 81001-5-1 standard) can help fulfill these obligations (e.g., encryption, user authentication, secure update mechanisms).

Prepare Technical Documentation (MDR Annex II)

The manufacturer must compile a comprehensive technical file demonstrating conformity. For SaMD, key contents are:

(a) Device description and specifications: An overview of the software, its intended medical purpose, target patient population, operating environment (e.g., mobile app, cloud service), and main functionalities. Include the software version and build, and describe any relevant hardware or accessories.

(b) Design and manufacturing information: Explanation of the software architecture and design (e.g., system block diagrams, data flow, algorithms used). Describe the development tools, programming languages, and the methods used for building and testing the software. Although "manufacturing" for software is intangible, this section covers the development lifecycle. If the software is distributed on hardware or through app stores, describe those processes.

(c) Risk management file: Complete documentation from the ISO 14971 process includes hazard identification, risk analysis, risk evaluation, risk control measures, and risk/benefit analysis. Each identified risk should be linked to mitigations and verification of those mitigations. This file demonstrates compliance with MDR's risk reduction requirements.

(d) Product verification and validation: All test reports and evidence demonstrating that the software fulfills its specifications and intended purpose. This includes software module/unit test results, integration test results, system testing (covering all functional requirements), and clinical validation results. For example, if the SaMD is an AI diagnostic tool, this section would include performance metrics on test datasets, comparisons to clinical gold standards, etc. The MDR requires evidence of analytical performance (does the software correctly perform its algorithm) and clinical performance (does using the software lead to the intended clinical outcome or decision). According to guidance, technical verification alone is insufficient for SaMD; clinical validation is also necessary.

(e) Clinical evaluation documentation: A Clinical Evaluation Report (CER) is required per MDR Article 61 and Annex XIV. This document synthesizes clinical evidence to demonstrate the device's safety and performance during actual use. For SaMD, the CER may include literature studies, results from clinical trials or field studies, and validation studies that compare the software's outputs to physician assessments or patient outcomes. MDCG 2020-1 states that the clinical evaluation of software can utilize derived data (e.g., from retrospective studies) but must ultimately demonstrate that the software's output is clinically accurate and provides a positive benefit-risk profile. The CER must conclude that the SaMD fulfills its intended purpose and is at least as effective as existing alternatives, if any.

(f) General Safety and Performance Requirements (GSPR) checklist: A mapping of how the device meets each applicable requirement in MDR Annex I. For instance, GSPR sections on chemical and electrical safety may be "not applicable" for pure software, but sections on clinical performance, risk controls, labeling, and cybersecurity will apply. Manufacturers usually reference standards (EN ISO or IEC) in this checklist to demonstrate compliance.

(g) Labeling: All information supplied with the device, including the Instructions for Use (IFU) and any labeling on a physical medium or download page. For SaMD, the IFU can be provided electronically. It must contain the necessary instructions, intended use, contraindications, warnings, etc., as per MDR Annex I (section 23). If the software is downloadable, the "label" might be the information on the app store or the accompanying user manual. Clear user guidance is especially important for SaMD to ensure correct use and awareness of any limitations.

The technical documentation must be systematically organized and readily accessible to the Notified Body. Frequent pitfalls that result in delays encompass absent components (e.g., lack of clinical data) or disorganized structure that hampers information retrieval. The BSI emphasizes that incomplete submissions and inadequately structured files frequently hinder review processes. Manufacturers are advised to ensure the technical file is thorough and internally coherent; for instance, assertions presented in the Instructions for Use (IFU) must be substantiated by corresponding validation evidence within the file.

Select Conformity Assessment Route and Notified Body Involvement
Depending on the class determined (per step 1), the regulatory route diverges:

(a) Class I (non-sterile, non-measuring) SaMD: The manufacturer can self-declare conformity. This involves preparing the technical documentation, complying with MDR, and drawing up a Declaration of Conformity. No Notified Body

(NB) review is required by law. However, under MDR's new Rule 11, very few SaMD remain Class I, so this scenario is rare (examples might be wellness apps that qualify as medical devices but with very minimal risk).

(b) Class IIa, IIb, or III Software as a Medical Device (SaMD): A conformity assessment by a Notified Body (NB) is required. The manufacturer must select an NB that is designated under the Medical Device Regulation (MDR) for the applicable device types, as several NBs currently encompass the scope for active devices, including software. The customary pathway involves MDR Annex IX, which encompasses Quality Management System (QMS) and Technical Documentation: the NB will conduct an audit of the manufacturer's QMS and evaluate the technical file. Alternatively, Annex X (Type Examination) in conjunction with Annex XI (Production Quality Assurance) may be adopted, although Annex IX is the more prevalent choice for software. Under Annex IX, Section I pertains to the QMS audit, while Section II relates to the assessment of the technical documentation for the device.

After selecting an NB and signing a contract, the conformity assessment process entails:

(a) NB Technical File Review: The NB's experts review the submitted documentation. They check each aspect for compliance with MDR. It's common for the NB to issue a list of questions or nonconformities if anything is unclear or insufficient. For example, they might ask for clarification on the clinical evaluation rationale, or request additional testing for a certain risk scenario. The manufacturer must respond with additional evidence or justifications. There may be multiple review cycles until all NB concerns are resolved. Efficient resolution of NB questions is key to avoiding delays.

(b) NB Quality System Audit: In parallel (or sometimes before/after tech file review), the NB conducts an on-site audit of the QMS. The audit verifies implementation of ISO 13485 principles: design control (ensure requirements trace to design outputs and validation), software development practices (per IEC 62304), supplier management (e.g., if using cloud services or open-source components, ensure controls are in place), complaint handling, etc. For initial MDR certification, this is typically a Stage 1 (readiness/document review) and Stage 2 (facility audit). If the company already has ISO 13485 certification, the NB may combine the audits. Any nonconformities found (e.g., missing risk management procedure, or inadequate testing documentation) must be corrected by the manufacturer and verified by NB before proceeding.

(c) Certification Decision: Once the technical documentation and Quality Management System (QMS) are determined to be compliant, the Notified Body (NB) issues an EU Quality Assurance Certificate (for the QMS) and an EU Technical Documentation Certificate, or a singular EU certificate encompassing both aspects as specified under Annex IX. This documentation essentially represents the CE certificate for the device. Consequently, the manufacturer concludes the EU Declaration of Conformity, thereby affirming that the device adheres to Medical Device Regulation (MDR) requirements. Subsequently, the CE mark may be affixed to the software (for instance, displayed in the software's "About" section or accompanying materials), allowing the device to be marketed throughout the European Union.

Post-Certification and Other Requirements

After obtaining CE marking, the manufacturer must fulfill MDR post-market obligations. This includes registering the device (and company) in EUDAMED (the European database), assigning a Unique Device Identification (UDI) code to the SaMD, and conducting Post-Market Surveillance (PMS). A Post-Market Clinical Follow-up (PMCF) plan may be part of the technical file, especially if the pre-market clinical evidence had gaps—the manufacturer will then collect real-world performance data to update the clinical evaluation over time. MDR also imposes vigilance duties: serious incidents or field safety corrective actions involving the software must be reported to authorities. These post-market activities, while outside the initial certification, are crucial for maintaining compliance and the CE mark validity (CE certificates under MDR have 5-year validity, with surveillance audits by NB annually or biannually in between).

Some Geographical Considerations

The certification of Software as a Medical Device (SaMD) within the European and German frameworks entails distinct approaches depending on the notified body (NB) or fast-track schemes involved. Below is a detailed narrative reconstruction of the comparative landscape, focusing on DiGA (Germany—BfArM), Kiwa (Netherlands/Italy), TÜV SÜD (Germany), and BSI (UK/NL).

DiGA (Germany)—BfArM Fast-Track

To qualify for the DiGA Fast-Track process, the Software as a Medical Device (SaMD) must possess a CE mark in accordance with the Medical Device Regulation (MDR), which is typically categorized as either a Class I or IIa medical device. The Federal Institute for Drugs and Medical Devices (BfArM) does not permit any exceptions regarding this requirement. The conformity assessment must be finalized, and the technical documentation must be prepared prior to submitting an application.

In addition to the prerequisite of a CE mark, BfArM mandates the submission of a specific application dossier that thoroughly addresses IT security, patient safety, data privacy (in compliance with the General Data Protection Regulation (GDPR) and the DiGAV 40-point checklist), as well as evidence of a favorable healthcare impact. This dossier must encompass not only the complete MDR technical file but also supplementary materials that illustrate the app's integration into the care pathway.

The requisites for clinical evidence are rigorous. A summary of a completed clinical evaluation is obligatory, along with a comprehensive outcomes study, which must demonstrate a measurable positive effect. Furthermore, the findings must be published within 1 year. For provisional listing, an ongoing study protocol may be submitted, with the expectation of full data delivery within a 12-month timeframe.

Regarding timelines, the DiGA process presents a distinct predictability: a maximum of three months from the moment the submission is acknowledged as complete, with no cessation of the timeline for clarification requests. This legal stipulation enables manufacturers to anticipate a decision (approval or rejection) within a narrow and reliable timeframe, contrasting with other Notified Body (NB) processes.

Risk management, while grounded in the MDR, is extended to encompass operational use scenarios. BfArM expects not only documentation of technical safety but also clearly defined mitigation strategies for real-world risks, such as user misinterpretation. Warning mechanisms, GDPR-compliant data management, and system-level security are scrutinized meticulously, often adhering to the guidelines provided by the British Standards Institution (BSI) on cybersecurity.

Concerning clinical effectiveness, the DiGA distinctly requires evidence of tangible improvements in care. This may include enhanced adherence, expedited recovery, or improved clinical outcomes directly attributable to the software. In situations where full evidence is not yet available, a provisional listing may be granted under the condition that robust data will be produced within a 12-month period. Transparency is mandated: the DiGA directory will indicate whether the positive effect has been substantiated or remains under investigation.

Kiwa (Netherlands/Italy)—MDR Notified Body

Kiwa acts as a traditional Notified Body under MDR (e.g., Kiwa Dare in the Netherlands or Kiwa Cermet in Italy), requiring a full Annex II technical file, which includes device description, GSPR checklist, verification and validation, and a complete clinical evaluation. They often supply guidance documents and accept submissions in English or Italian, with emphasis on clear executive summaries.

Kiwa places value on standard compliance (ISO 14971, IEC 62304) and expects that software development documentation aligns with lifecycle expectations. Their scope includes active devices and software, and therefore their reviews are adapted to SaMD-specific characteristics.

Timelines are moderate, usually ranging from 6 to 12 months depending on documentation completeness and audit scheduling. Kiwa's review may complete closer to 6 months for highly prepared submissions but can extend toward a year if multiple rounds of clarification are needed.

Their approach to risk management is pragmatic. As long as a thorough ISO 14971-compliant risk analysis is presented and risks are mitigated or transparently communicated (e.g., via labeling), Kiwa generally avoids overly conservative interpretations. They are not known for being bureaucratic, and auditors are regarded as practical and reasonable.

In clinical evaluation, Kiwa adheres to MDR expectations but is flexible. For low-risk devices, literature-based Clinical Evaluation Reports (CERs) or bench testing might suffice. For higher-risk or novel software, clinical performance data is essential. They follow MDCG guidance for equivalence justifications and accept proportionate evidence rather than imposing excessive requirements.

TÜV SÜD (Germany)—MDR Notified Body

TÜV SÜD is renowned for its meticulous technical scrutiny. The Notified Body (NB) mandates comprehensive Medical Device Regulation (MDR) documentation and frequently requests supplementary materials such as traceability matrices or software architecture diagrams. Submissions are anticipated in well-organized formats (e.g., bookmarked PDFs), with the assignment of a reviewer specializing in software.

The review process of TÜV SÜD encompasses significant emphasis on software validation, algorithm transparency, and cybersecurity. Should artificial intelligence (AI) be involved, TÜV SÜD may request a validation methodology that addresses bias, retraining, and dataset integrity, even in instances where it is not explicitly mandated by the MDR.

The timeline established by TÜV SÜD tends to be extensive, typically spanning from 9 to 12 months or more. Although expedited review options are available, access to these services is limited and contingent upon resource availability. Companies frequently select TÜV SÜD due to its esteemed reputation, particularly when aiming for markets where stringent certification is regarded as a key differentiator.

Risk management protocols at TÜV SÜD are stringent yet methodical. Auditors anticipate comprehensive hazard identification, mitigation strategies, and validation processes. Low-probability risks with high severity are not overlooked; instead, TÜV SÜD may request fallback mechanisms, robust testing, and justifications that extend beyond mere labeling. Their underlying philosophy promotes inherent safety by design.

With respect to clinical data, TÜV SÜD expects a robust evidential foundation, particularly when diagnostic claims are asserted. The Clinical Evaluation Reports (CERs) undergo rigorous scrutiny, and there is often a preference for real-world clinical data over simulated scenarios. For novel devices, this may escalate to expectations akin to premarket clinical trials. Furthermore, post-market follow-up may be mandated if initial evidence reveals deficiencies.

BSI (UK/NL)—MDR Notified Body

The British Standards Institution (BSI) offers structured guidance for Medical Device Regulation (MDR) submissions and has published best practices to support manufacturers. BSI requires comprehensive MDR documentation, accompanied by an explanatory cover letter and, frequently, a structured summary of clinical evidence.

Generally, BSI adheres to the MDR requirements without imposing additional documentation demands; however, individual auditors may examine specific issues in greater depth. The BSI team possesses specialized expertise in software and artificial intelligence and has adopted emerging international guidelines, such as those outlined by the International Medical Device Regulators Forum (IMDRF).

Timelines for BSI's processes vary. Initial reviews can commence within 2–3 months, and well-prepared submissions may result in CE certification within approximately 6 months. In contrast, complex or iterative reviews may prolong the timelines to between 9 and 12 months. Although BSI is capable of processing documents in parallel, the outcomes are significantly influenced by the reviewing team involved.

Risk management reviews conducted by BSI are noted to be inconsistent. While some auditors demonstrate clarity and structure, others may focus on minor risks or necessitate highly detailed justifications. Nonetheless, compliance with ISO 14971 and a robust benefit-risk analysis remain imperative. Cybersecurity considerations are routinely assessed.

From a clinical perspective, BSI requires substantial evidence that is in alignment with the MDR. However, there are instances when BSI may request more extensive data than analogous organizations, even for products with established precedents. For example, user studies may be requested to confirm appropriate usage, or additional literature may be required for diagnostic algorithms. BSI emphasizes the need to validate claims with scientific rigor and may necessitate post-market studies to corroborate performance should pre-market data be insufficient.

This comprehensive overview, as summarized in Table D.1 below, delineates the key differences in regulatory expectations among various schemes and bodies. While DiGA prioritizes speed, transparency, and clinical benefit, Notified Bodies such as TÜV SÜD and BSI tend to emphasize methodological rigor and

Table D.1 Regulatory comparison table for SaMD certification

Notified body/ scheme	Documentation requirements	Average timeline	Risk management approach	Clinical evidence approach
DiGA (Germany)—BfArM Fast-Track	Prerequisite: CE Mark under MDR	~3 months (fixed by law)	CE-based plus real-world safety measures	Requires study showing positive care effect
	Additional application dossier covering data privacy, IT security, patient safety, and positive healthcare effect		Context-specific warnings required	Allows provisional listing with study commitment
	Clinical study documentation with summary and commitment to publish.		Focus on GDPR and cybersecurity compliance.	Evidence must show real-world benefits.

(continued)

Table D.1 (continued)

Notified body/ scheme	Documentation requirements	Average timeline	Risk management approach	Clinical evidence approach
Kiwa (Netherlands/ Italy)—MDR NB	Standard MDR Technical File	~6–12 months	ISO 14971 compliance verified	MDR-compliant CER
	Templates/checklists often provided		Pragmatic, not overly conservative	Literature-based or usability studies accepted for low-risk
	Strong emphasis on standards (ISO 14971, IEC 62304)		Accepts reasonable controls and justifications	Clinical data needed for novel/critical software
TÜV SÜD (Germany)—MDR NB	Full MDR documentation plus detailed supporting documents	9+ months	Very stringent, risk-benefit analysis required	High bar: requires robust clinical performance data
	Strong focus on software architecture and validation		Verifies mitigations and tests	Prefers real-world or clinical trial data
	Software specialist auditors assigned		Inherent safety preferred over labeling.	PMCF may be required.
BSI (UK/ NL)—MDR NB	Full MDR documentation	6–12 months	Varies by auditor	Aligned with MDR but occasionally more demanding
	Requests clear documentation with summaries		Thorough ISO 14971 process	Requires strong correlation between software output and clinical outcomes
	May include best practice guides and specific formats for clinical evidence		Strong emphasis on benefit-risk analysis and cybersecurity	May request user studies or additional literature

conservative interpretations of risk and evidence. In contrast, Kiwa adopts a pragmatic and proportionate approach that is grounded in the Medical Device Regulation (MDR) but manifests a more streamlined attitude.

Post-Certification and Other Requirements

After obtaining CE marking, the manufacturer must fulfill MDR post-market obligations. This includes registering the device (and company) in EUDAMED (the European database), assigning a Unique Device Identification (UDI) code to the SaMD, and conducting Post-Market Surveillance (PMS). A Post-Market Clinical

Follow-up (PMCF) plan may be part of the technical file, especially if the pre-market clinical evidence had gaps—the manufacturer will then collect real-world performance data to update the clinical evaluation over time. MDR also imposes vigilance duties: serious incidents or field safety corrective actions involving the software must be reported to authorities. These post-market activities, while outside the initial certification, are crucial for maintaining compliance and the CE mark validity (CE certificates under MDR have 5-year validity, with surveillance audits by NB annually or biannually in between).

In summary, the conformity assessment for SaMD under MDR is comprehensive. It mirrors the process for other medical devices, with special attention to the software lifecycle and clinical validation. Key normative references like ISO 13485, ISO 14971, and IEC 62304 are essential to meet MDR's state-of-the-art requirements in documentation. Compared to pre-2021 (MDD regime), MDR demands more robust evidence (particularly clinical) and formalized documentation. Manufacturers often find the MDR process similar to an FDA submission in rigor, with some noting the EU route has become more structured and "FDA-like" in requiring detailed proof of safety and performance. Proper planning, including early risk classification, QMS implementation, and gathering clinical evidence, can smooth the path. Typically, expect around 6–12 months from the start of the NB application to the CE certificate for a well-prepared SaMD submission, although timing varies widely. In some cases, resource constraints in NBs have pushed timelines beyond a year, so engaging with the NB early and ensuring a complete submission is critical.

Procedural Comparison: European Notified Bodies and the DiGA Fast-Track

While the requirements of the Medical Device Regulation (MDR) are standardized, different European Notified Bodies (NBs) may exhibit varying processes, areas of expertise, and turnaround times in the certification of Software as a Medical Device (SaMD). Furthermore, Germany's Digital Health Applications (DiGA) fast-track program, which is administered by the Federal Institute for Drugs and Medical Devices (BfArM), represents a distinct procedure for digital health applications following CE marking. In the following section, we conduct a comparative analysis of the procedures adopted by selected Notified Bodies, namely, Kiwa (NL/IT), TÜV SÜD (DE), and BSI (UK/NL), as well as the DiGA process. This comparison emphasizes documentation requirements, average assessment timelines, risk management approaches, and expectations regarding clinical evidence.

Note: Other Notified Bodies (NBs) with Software as a Medical Device (SaMD) experience include Dekra (DE), DQS Medizinprodukte (DE), SGS (BE), GMED (FR), among others. Some industry experts recommend considering less crowded NBs. For instance, DQS or Berlin Cert have been cited as possessing auditors with a robust understanding of software and more reasonable responsiveness. The selection of a Notified Body can significantly influence the regulatory journey: larger NBs (such as BSI and TÜV) provide extensive expertise but impose heavier demands, while smaller NBs may offer greater agility and enhanced communication. Regardless of the chosen Notified Body, aligning with the Medical Device Regulation (MDR) requirements remains the consistent factor for success.

Conclusion

We have conducted a comprehensive analysis of how MDR 2017/745 is applicable to Software as a Medical Device and the prerequisites for obtaining CE certification. The significant findings indicate a more stringent risk classification (Rule 11), which categorizes the majority of SaMD into Class II or III, necessitating oversight from a Notified Body. Furthermore, the process of conformity assessment is methodical and involves the establishment of a robust Quality Management System (QMS), the preparation of extensive technical documentation, and the demonstration of safety and performance, frequently achieved through clinical evidence. Moreover, we have compared the procedures among various Notified Bodies and Germany's Digital Health Applications (DiGA) scheme, emphasizing disparities in documentation requirements, timelines, risk assessment philosophies, and evidence stipulations. Although the Medical Device Regulation (MDR) sets a standardized regulatory benchmark, manufacturers must remain cognizant of these practical variations. For instance, one Notified Body may expedite the process but pose atypical inquiries, while another may adopt a slower yet highly systematic approach, and the DiGA mandates evidence of real-world benefits that extend beyond mere compliance.

For manufacturers of Software as a Medical Device (SaMD), the process of obtaining CE marking under the Medical Device Regulation (MDR) can prove to be both challenging and resource-intensive. Nevertheless, comprehensive preparation—such as the implementation of standards like ISO 13485, ISO 14971, and IEC 62304, along with meticulous compilation of all required evidence—will significantly streamline the review process. The selection of an appropriate Notified Body, alongside early engagement through pre-submission meetings when feasible, is also a strategic consideration. In markets such as Germany, it is crucial to plan for post-market evaluation schemes like the Digital Healthcare Act (DiGA) if the product aims to secure reimbursement, as this introduces additional requirements, particularly concerning clinical effectiveness.

In conclusion, MDR 2017/745 has established a new benchmark for Software as a Medical Device (SaMD) certification. By comprehending the regulations and the expectations of Notified Bodies, developers can proficiently navigate the certifying process. This bilingual report, which includes clearly defined headings and a comparative table, endeavors to assist stakeholders in both understanding the regulatory requirements and strategically planning for SaMD CE compliance in Europe.

Appendix E: Glossary of Key Terms

1. *P4 Medicine:* A healthcare model focused on four key principles:
   Predictive: Leveraging data and analytics to anticipate health issues.
   Preventive: Using insights to reduce the likelihood of disease.

Personalized: Tailoring care to the individual needs of each patient.
Participatory: Encouraging patients to take an active role in their health management.

2. *Adaptive Treatment:* A dynamic approach to patient care where therapies are adjusted in real-time based on patient response, facilitated by tools like predictive analytics and biomarkers.
3. *Artificial Intelligence (AI):* The use of algorithms and machine learning to process data, identify patterns, and support clinical decision-making in areas such as diagnostics, treatment planning, and operational workflows.
4. *Augmented Reality (AR):* Technology that overlays digital visuals or information onto the physical world is employed in healthcare for surgical training, patient education, and therapy.
5. *Big Data:* Extremely large datasets collected from diverse sources, such as EHRs, wearables, and genomics, are analyzed to generate insights for individual and population health management.
6. *Bioelectronic Medicine:* Electronic devices such as implantable neurostimulators or wearable biosensors are used to interface with biological systems for monitoring or treating diseases.
7. *Change Management:* Structured strategies and processes used to help organizations transition from traditional to digital workflows, fostering acceptance and adoption among staff.
8. *Clinical Decision Support Systems (cDSS):* Digital tools that analyze data and provide clinicians with evidence-based recommendations to enhance decision-making.
9. *Continuous Care:* A model of healthcare delivery that provides ongoing monitoring and support, moving away from episodic interventions to continuous engagement with patients.
10. *Data Governance:* Policies and practices ensuring that data is collected, stored, shared, and used responsibly, maintaining compliance with regulations like GDPR and HIPAA.
11. *Digital Therapeutics (DTx)*: Software-based treatments that provide therapeutic interventions for medical conditions, often validated through clinical trials and regulated like traditional medical devices.
12. *Electronic Health Record (EHR):* A digital platform for storing patient health information, facilitating communication and data exchange among healthcare providers.
13. *Explainable AI (XAI):* Artificial intelligence systems designed to provide transparent and interpretable outputs, ensuring that clinicians and patients understand how decisions are made.
14. *Gamification:* The integration of game-like elements, such as rewards and challenges, into Digital Health tools to motivate behavior change and improve adherence to care plans.

15. *Health Data Interoperability:* The ability of different health systems, devices, and platforms to exchange, interpret, and use patient data seamlessly.
16. *mHealth (Mobile Health):* The use of mobile devices, such as smartphones and tablets, to deliver healthcare services, manage chronic conditions, and promote wellness.
17. *Neural Interfaces*: Technologies that connect the nervous system to electronic devices, enabling applications like brain–computer interfaces or neurostimulation.
18. *Predictive Analytics:* Techniques that analyze historical and real-time data to forecast future outcomes, enabling proactive care and resource allocation.
19. *Precision Medicine:* A healthcare approach that considers individual genetic, environmental, and lifestyle factors to develop tailored treatment plans.
20. *Privacy-by-Design:* A principle ensuring that privacy measures are integrated into digital tools and processes from the outset rather than added as an afterthought.
21. *Remote Patient Monitoring (RPM):* The use of digital devices to collect health data outside clinical settings, such as at home, and transmit it to healthcare providers for analysis.
22. *Software as a Medical Device (SaMD):* Software that performs medical functions, such as diagnosing conditions or managing treatment plans, often regulated as a medical device.
23. *Telehealth:* A broad term encompassing the remote delivery of healthcare services and information, including telemedicine, remote monitoring, and health education.
24. *Telemedicine:* The use of video conferencing, phone calls, or online platforms for real-time consultations between patients and healthcare providers.
25. *Value-Based Care:* A healthcare payment model that incentivises providers based on patient outcomes rather than the volume of services delivered.
26. *Virtual Reality (VR):* Fully immersive digital environments are used in healthcare for medical training, pain management, and therapeutic interventions.
27. *Wearables:* Devices worn on the body, such as smartwatches or fitness trackers, monitor health metrics and provide real-time feedback to users and healthcare providers.
28. *Wellness:* A proactive approach to health management focused on prevention, lifestyle optimization, and overall well-being rather than merely treating illness.
29. *European Health Data Space (EHDS):* A regulatory framework aimed at enabling secure, standardized sharing of health data across European Union member states to improve care and foster innovation.
30. *Data Altruism*: This concept, introduced in the European Data Governance Act, involves individuals voluntarily sharing anonymised data for the public good, such as research or public health initiatives.

Appendix F: Practical Resources for Digital Medicine

Summaries of Key Regulations and Compliance Frameworks

Understanding the regulatory landscape is crucial for the safe and effective implementation of Digital Medicine. Below are brief overviews of the most relevant regulatory frameworks:

General Data Protection Regulation (GDPR)—EU

The GDPR (Regulation (EU) 2016/679) is a comprehensive privacy and security framework that governs personal data protection in the European Union.

It affects Digital Medicine by defining patient data as "sensitive" and necessitating explicit consent for collection and processing; mandating data minimization, encryption, and pseudonymization to safeguard patient privacy; and ensuring patients' right to access, correct, and delete their health data (Right to Be Forgotten).

Relevance to Digital Medicine: Any digital health platform operating in Europe—whether telemedicine, AI-driven diagnostics, or remote monitoring—must comply with GDPR's stringent security and consent requirements.

Health Insurance Portability and Accountability Act (HIPAA)—US

HIPAA (1996, updated via the HITECH Act of 2009) is the primary legislation in the US governing the privacy and security of health data. It mandates stringent safeguards for Protected Health Information (PHI), ensuring secure storage, transmission, and sharing; Business Associate Agreements (BAAs) for digital health vendors handling PHI (e.g., cloud storage providers and AI analytics platforms); and breach notification rules in the event of data leaks, guaranteeing patient awareness and regulatory action.

Relevance to Digital Medicine: any digital tool used in the US healthcare system (e.g., AI-powered EHRs, telehealth apps) must comply with HIPAA to avoid penalties and ensure patient trust.

FDA Digital Health Policies—US

The US Food and Drug Administration (FDA) regulates Digital Medicine tools under its Software as a Medical Device (SaMD) framework. It categorizes digital solutions into low-risk wellness tools (e.g., step counters, and general fitness apps) that do not require FDA approval; moderate-risk medical software (e.g., AI-based ECG analysis, and digital therapeutics) that require clinical validation and regulatory approval; and high-risk AI-powered diagnostics (e.g., autonomous radiology AI) that are subject to pre-market review and continuous post-market surveillance.

Relevance to Digital Medicine: Developers of clinical-grade AI tools and digital therapeutics must navigate FDA clearance pathways (e.g., 510(k), De Novo, or PMA) to ensure patient safety.

European Health Data Space (EHDS)—EU Regulation

The *European Health Data Space (EHDS)* is a EU initiative that aims to facilitate the secure cross-border sharing of health data. Its primary objectives include enabling patients to access and manage their medical records across EU member states, advocating for the secondary use of anonymized health data for research and innovation, and ensuring the interoperability and standardization of electronic health records (EHRs) throughout Europe.

Future Impact on Digital Medicine: EHDS will play a pivotal role in harmonizing digital health regulations across the EU, fostering innovation while protecting privacy.

Evaluation Checklists and Implementation Blueprints

These checklists provide structured methodologies for assessing digital tools before clinical adoption.

Digital Health Assessment Framework

Before integrating a digital health solution into practice, healthcare organizations should evaluate:

Clinical Validation: Is the tool supported by peer-reviewed evidence or clinical trials? Has it received regulatory approval (FDA, MDR, or equivalent)?

Data Security & Compliance: Does it comply with GDPR/HIPAA? Are data encrypted in transit and at rest? Is patient consent clearly defined?

Interoperability & Integration: Does it integrate with existing EHR systems (HL7 FHIR, DICOM)? Can it exchange data securely with other health IT platforms?

User Experience & Engagement: Is the tool clinician-friendly with minimal workflow disruption?

Does it provide clear, actionable insights rather than overwhelming users with data?

Implementation Blueprint for Digital Medicine Solutions

When rolling out a new digital tool, follow this structured approach:

Step 1: Define Clinical and Operational Goals: What problem does this technology address? (e.g., reducing readmissions, enhancing diagnostics); how will success be evaluated? (KPIs: patient outcomes, cost savings, workflow efficiency)

Step 2: Engage Key Stakeholders Early: involve clinicians, administrators, and IT teams from the outset; address potential resistance to adoption through education and training.

Step 3: Conduct a Small-Scale Pilot; test the solution in a controlled setting before full deployment;

Collect feedback from early adopters to enhance usability.

Step 4: Scale Up with Continuous Monitoring; integrate with EHRs and other clinical systems; monitor performance through real-world data analytics; ensure sustained compliance with privacy and security regulations.

Recommended Reading and Additional Resources

Artificial Intelligence & Digital Health: Key References

As AI-driven healthcare solutions gain momentum, clinicians, administrators, and policymakers must comprehend their implications, applications, and ethical considerations. Below is a comprehensive collection of books, reports, and peer-reviewed articles examining AI's role in Digital Medicine.

Books and Reports

Topol, E. (2019). *Deep Medicine: How Artificial Intelligence Can Make Healthcare Human Again.* Basic Books.

A seminal work that explores AI's potential to enhance clinical decision-making while restoring humanistic medicine.

Specialty-Specific Action Plans and Checklists for Digital Medicine Integration

Introduction

Digital medicine is not a one-size-fits-all paradigm. Each medical specialty operates within unique clinical, operational, and regulatory boundaries. This appendix provides tailored checklists and structured action plans to help clinicians, administrators, and innovators align digital tools with the specific needs of their specialty. Whether for early pilots or at-scale implementation, these frameworks offer practical pathways toward effective, equitable, and sustainable integration.

Cardiology

Focus: Remote Monitoring, AI-Driven Risk Stratification, Digital Therapeutics for Heart Failure

Checklist

1. Evaluate current use of wearables and RPM for chronic heart failure (CHF): These technologies can detect early signs of decompensation and reduce avoidable hospitalizations.
2. Identify validated DTx platforms for post-MI or hypertension management: Digital therapeutics offer structured interventions that can support adherence and lifestyle modification.
3. Establish data-sharing protocols with cardiology imaging (e.g., AI echocardiography): Interoperable systems allow for more integrated and timely care.

4. Ensure EHR integration with ECG and rhythm monitoring apps: Continuous data flow from devices supports proactive care.
5. Train staff on alert fatigue management for digital alerts (AF, VT detection): Managing false positives and thresholds is essential to maintain clinical trust.

Action Plan

- Phase 1: Pilot ECG-capable wearables in high-risk CHF patients with structured feedback loops.
- Phase 2: Integrate AI-based risk stratification tools in outpatient cardiology workflows.
- Phase 3: Introduce DTx platforms for hypertension and CHF with real-world outcome tracking.

Endocrinology/Diabetology

Focus: Continuous Glucose Monitoring (CGM), Mobile Coaching, SaMDs for Type 1 and 2 DM

Checklist

1. Assess access to CGM among T1D and insulin-treated T2D patients: Identify disparities and reimbursement barriers.
2. Evaluate use of SaMDs for insulin titration or lifestyle coaching: These can reduce hypo/hyperglycemia risk and empower patient self-management.
3. Verify compliance with MDR for digital insulin management platforms: Compliance with regulation ensures safe deployment.
4. Analyze real-world data integration with labs and pharmacies: Interoperability supports a closed-loop feedback system.
5. Monitor outcomes through validated PROMs (e.g., DDS or WHO-5): Ensures a patient-centered evaluation of digital tools.

Action Plan

- Phase 1: Integrate CGM dashboards into endocrinology visits.
- Phase 2: Train diabetes educators in coaching models augmented by mobile apps.
- Phase 3: Collaborate with national diabetes registries to capture digital outcomes.

Oncology

Focus: Symptom Tracking, Precision Medicine Dashboards, Survivorship Support

Checklist

1. Implement patient-reported outcome (PRO) systems for treatment monitoring: Enables real-time management of toxicities and adherence.
2. Use digital tools for symptom side-effect management (e.g., fatigue, mucositis): Supports personalized care during chemotherapy.
3. Integrate molecular diagnostics with digital dashboards: Aligns treatment decisions with genomic profiles.

4. Ensure GDPR and GCP compliance of oncology-focused platforms: Particularly critical for trials and longitudinal tracking.
5. Deploy survivorship apps with secure patient access: Empower patients during follow-up phases.

Action Plan

- Phase 1: Launch digital PRO tracking for chemotherapy patients.
- Phase 2: Connect tumor boards with AI-assisted clinical decision tools.
- Phase 3: Scale survivorship apps for follow-up and quality-of-life monitoring.

Psychiatry and Mental Health

Focus: Digital CBT, Mobile Screening Tools, AI-Enabled Triage

Checklist

1. Introduce app-based CBT with CE/FDA clearance: Effective for mild to moderate anxiety and depression.
2. Develop clear referral pathways to blended digital therapy: Hybrid models are more sustainable.
3. Train clinicians to prescribe and monitor digital mental health tools: Increases digital confidence and patient trust.
4. Use AI chatbots or speech analysis tools for early detection: Ideal for triage or support in under-resourced areas.
5. Prioritize ethical compliance and informed consent, especially with minors: Mental health data is among the most sensitive.

Action Plan

- Phase 1: Offer app-based CBT in mental health clinics.
- Phase 2: Use AI-driven chat tools for triage in community settings.
- Phase 3: Embed long-term support systems using mobile engagement platforms.

Primary Care/Family Medicine

Focus: Digital Triage, Chronic Care Management, Patient Engagement

Checklist

1. Implement digital symptom checkers for triage: Reduces unnecessary visits and helps prioritize care.
2. Facilitate digital communication with patients (chat, video, secure portals): Enhances access while respecting workloads.
3. Track multiple chronic conditions through a digital dashboard: Supports holistic care, particularly in multimorbidity.
4. Align digital tools with national or regional digital formularies: Enables reimbursement and compliance.
5. Promote digital literacy campaigns in the patient population: Mitigates the digital divide.

Action Plan

- Phase 1: Introduce pre-visit symptom checkers.
- Phase 2: Deploy remote monitoring for hypertension and diabetes.
- Phase 3: Embed digital coaching into annual check-up programs.

Pediatrics

Focus: mHealth for Parents, Chronic Care in Children, Digital Developmental Screening

Checklist

1. Adopt teleconsultation platforms designed for pediatric needs: Privacy, consent, and simplicity must be built-in.
2. Use gamified apps to support treatment adherence (e.g., asthma, ADHD): Playful approaches boost engagement.
3. Ensure consent processes are clear and age-appropriate: Essential when working with minors.
4. Integrate school and community feedback in digital care: Enables holistic support.
5. Limit digital overload in younger children: Balance screen time with therapeutic value.

Action Plan

- Phase 1: Initiate telepediatrics for asthma, epilepsy, ADHD.
- Phase 2: Use digital diaries and gamified interventions in chronic care.
- Phase 3: Collaborate with schools to embed mHealth in health education.

Neurology

Focus: Epilepsy Monitoring, Cognitive Screening, Stroke Rehab

Checklist

1. Introduce wearable EEG and seizure detection tools: Enhance monitoring for epilepsy patients in outpatient settings.
2. Adopt digital rehab platforms with motion sensors and AI: Optimize stroke recovery at home.
3. Pilot cognitive screening tools for early dementia detection: Cost-effective and scalable in aging populations.
4. Ensure seamless integration with neuroimaging and records: Improves coordination and reduces redundancy.
5. Design tools for cognitive or motor impairment accessibility: Usability is paramount in neurological populations.

Action Plan

- Phase 1: Launch seizure monitoring pilots in epilepsy clinics.
- Phase 2: Deploy telerehab platforms in poststroke care.
- Phase 3: Develop cognitive screening pathways using validated mobile tools.

Rheumatology

Focus: Remote Disease Monitoring, Adherence Support, Digital PROs

Checklist

1. Use app-based flare and pain diaries: Helps track disease activity in RA or PsA.
2. Introduce digital joint assessment tools (e.g., AI movement tracking): Augments clinical evaluation remotely.
3. Monitor medication adherence with app reminders: Prevents treatment lapses.
4. Ensure connection to biologics registries for real-world data: Facilitates outcome research.
5. Mitigate digital fatigue in chronic patients: Use simplified interfaces and low-burden tools.

Action Plan

- Phase 1: Distribute symptom-logging tools in rheumatology clinics.
- Phase 2: Enable remote assessments during teleconsultations.
- Phase 3: Build data-sharing agreements with pharma and registries.

Infectious Diseases

Focus: Outbreak Monitoring, Digital DOT, AI for Epidemiology

Checklist

1. Test mobile DOT for TB/HIV adherence: Reduces the need for in-person observation.
2. Deploy AI dashboards to monitor nosocomial infections: Early alerts prevent spread.
3. Integrate geolocation tracing tools in public health: Must comply with privacy laws.
4. Use SMS/mApp-based symptom tracking during outbreaks: Real-time public health data.
5. Monitor ethical implications of digital surveillance: Especially under emergency declarations.

Action Plan

- Phase 1: Launch digital adherence pilots in TB and HIV care.
- Phase 2: Roll out infection analytics tools in hospital infection control units.
- Phase 3: Collaborate with public health agencies to scale outbreak monitoring tools.

Pulmonology

Focus: COPD/Asthma Remote Management, Sleep Disorder Screening, Air Quality Alerts

Checklist

1. Introduce connected inhalers for adherence and usage tracking: Empowers patients and clinicians.

2. Use remote spirometry and peak flow sensors: Supports monitoring in between visits.
3. Adopt digital sleep assessment tools for sleep apnea: Reduces underdiagnosis.
4. Provide environmental trigger alerts to patients: Enhances self-care.
5. Train care teams on device support and patient coaching: Improves long-term engagement.

Action Plan
- Phase 1: Distribute connected devices for asthma/COPD.
- Phase 2: Implement digital screening pathways for sleep apnea.
- Phase 3: Use personalized environmental data in action plans.

Rehabilitation Medicine

Focus: Telerehab, Motion Sensors, Gamification

Checklist
1. Use video-based supervised rehab platforms: Ensures real-time correction and motivation.
2. Integrate wearables to track gait, posture, strength: Enables feedback outside of clinic.
3. Adopt gamified solutions to increase adherence: Especially valuable in younger or tech-savvy populations.
4. Streamline reporting into rehab documentation systems: Avoid double documentation.
5. Assess usability and satisfaction regularly: Improves engagement and outcomes.

Action Plan
- Phase 1: Pilot virtual rehab sessions post-surgery.
- Phase 2: Introduce sensor-based movement monitoring.
- Phase 3: Expand gamified rehab for arthritis, stroke, and musculoskeletal conditions.

Dermatology

Focus: AI Image Analysis, Remote Consults, Chronic Skin Conditions

Checklist
1. Evaluate AI tools for lesion classification: Supports triage and melanoma detection.
2. Expand teledermatology for rural access: Asynchronous image review is efficient.
3. Ensure quality in patient-submitted photos: Lighting, resolution, and consent are key.
4. Use digital platforms for eczema, psoriasis follow-up: Track flares and response to treatment.
5. Train GPs to use digital triage before referrals: Streamlines specialist pathways.

Action Plan

- Phase 1: Launch AI-assisted lesion screening in primary care.
- Phase 2: Enable remote consults through secure image upload.
- Phase 3: Use apps for chronic dermatologic conditions with patient-reported tracking.

Geriatrics

Focus: Frailty Monitoring, Polypharmacy Management, Digital Inclusion

Checklist

1. Introduce frailty screening tools integrated with EHRs: Tools such as the eFI (electronic Frailty Index) can help stratify risk early in care planning.
2. Implement medication reconciliation tools for polypharmacy: Digital tools can flag potential drug interactions, duplications, or deprescribing opportunities.
3. Facilitate remote monitoring of falls, vitals, and activity: Wearables or ambient sensors can support home-based aging.
4. Ensure digital tools are adapted for visual, cognitive, or motor impairments: Simple interfaces, voice support, and large fonts are essential.
5. Promote digital literacy and inclusion in older adults: Combine digital interventions with training or caregiver support.

Action Plan

- Phase 1: Deploy frailty screening in primary and community care settings.
- Phase 2: Use medication management platforms in nursing homes and geriatrics wards.
- Phase 3: Launch remote monitoring pilots for fall detection and early warning signs of decline.

Nephrology

Focus: CKD Monitoring, Dialysis Support, AI Risk Stratification

Checklist

1. Use mobile platforms to monitor weight, fluid status, and BP in CKD patients: Early signs of decompensation can be captured remotely.
2. Digitize dialysis logs and adherence tracking: Both home and in-center dialysis benefit from structured digital monitoring.
3. Apply AI tools for progression prediction in CKD: Machine learning can support early referral to nephrology.
4. Ensure interoperability with lab systems (e.g., creatinine, GFR, albumin): Data flow from external labs to nephrology dashboards enhances longitudinal tracking.
5. Enable patient engagement tools in pre-dialysis education: Digital education supports shared decision-making.

Action Plan

- Phase 1: Roll out self-monitoring apps for stage 3-4 CKD patients.
- Phase 2: Integrate AI risk models to predict CKD-to-ESRD progression.
- Phase 3: Use digital tools for home dialysis adherence and remote coaching.

Gastroenterology/Hepatology

Focus: IBD Symptom Tracking, Cirrhosis Monitoring, Digital Nutrition Support

Checklist

1. Deploy IBD patient apps for tracking flares, stools, and diet: These help in optimizing therapy and detecting relapses early.
2. Use wearables for ascites and weight monitoring in cirrhotic patients: Enables early identification of fluid overload.
3. Enable AI-driven reading of capsule endoscopy and pathology: Supports efficiency in diagnostic workflows.
4. Embed dietary coaching and nutrition tracking into chronic care: Especially important in hepatic steatosis, Crohn's disease, and post-op patients.
5. Monitor mental health comorbidities (e.g., anxiety in IBD): Integrated tools can support psychosomatic well-being.

Action Plan

- Phase 1: Pilot IBD tracking apps for flare detection and patient self-reporting.
- Phase 2: Introduce remote monitoring for cirrhosis with real-time alerts.
- Phase 3: Launch digital dietary support integrated with teleconsults.

Surgery (General and Specialized)

Focus: Prehabilitation, Remote Recovery Monitoring, Digital Consent

Checklist

1. Introduce preoperative digital screening and preparation platforms: These help optimize surgical readiness, especially in elderly or comorbid patients.
2. Use tele-follow-up platforms post-discharge for wound checks and pain tracking: Reduces readmissions and enables early intervention.
3. Adopt remote tools for rehabilitation and exercise tracking after surgery: Ensures patients recover functionality while reducing clinic visits.
4. Ensure digital consent platforms meet medico-legal standards: Video and electronic consent can improve comprehension and documentation.
5. Monitor PROMs to assess surgical recovery: Tools like QoR-15 or functional scores support patient-centered outcomes.

Action Plan

- Phase 1: Deploy pre-op digital pathways for elective surgeries (cardiac, ortho, abdominal).
- Phase 2: Use digital follow-up tools with wound image sharing and symptom alerts.
- Phase 3: Integrate post-op rehab apps and measure recovery with structured digital PROMs.

Closing Note

This appendix is not exhaustive but offers a dynamic framework for specialty-specific digital medicine planning. Clinical leaders are encouraged to revisit and update these checklists regularly based on regulatory evolutions, patient needs, and technology advancements.

References

Appendix A

Agentic Artificial Intelligence

1. Zou J, Topol EJ. The rise of agentic AI teammates in medicine. The Lancet. 2025;405(10477):457. https://doi.org/10.1016/S0140-6736(25)00202-8.
2. Hinostroza Fuentes VG, Abdul Karim H, Tan MJT, AlDahoul N. AI with agency: a vision for adaptive, efficient, and ethical healthcare. Front Digit Health. 2025;7 https://doi.org/10.3389/fdgth.2025.1600216.
3. Lakhan SE. The agentic era: why biopharma must embrace artificial intelligence that acts, not just informs. Cureus. 2025;17(5):e83390. https://doi.org/10.7759/cureus.83390.
4. Singh A. Agentic AI in healthcare: diagnosis and treatment (Working paper). SSRN; 2025. https://doi.org/10.2139/ssrn.5214492.

Blockchain in Digital Medicine

5. Vervoort D, Guetter CR, Peters AW. Blockchain, health disparities and global health. BMJ Innov. 2021;7(2):506–14. https://doi.org/10.1136/bmjinnov-2021-000667.
6. Kasyapa MSB, Vanmathi C. Blockchain integration in healthcare: a comprehensive investigation of use cases, performance issues, and mitigation strategies. Front Digit Health. 2024;6 https://doi.org/10.3389/fdgth.2024.1359858.
7. Bakrin FS, Tan CS, Goh KW, et al. The use of blockchain technology in the health care sector: systematic review. JMIR Med Informatics. 2022;10(1):e17278. https://doi.org/10.2196/17278.
8. EU Blockchain Observatory and Forum. Blockchain applications in the healthcare sector (Thematic report). European Commission; 2022. Retrieved from https://www.eublockchainforum.eu/ (February 8, 2022).

A. Cesario et al., *Digital Medicine Starter Guide*,
https://doi.org/10.1007/978-3-032-01272-2

Quantum Computing in Digital Medicine

9. Qayyum A, Ur Rasool R, Ahmad HF, Rafique W, Qadir J, Anwar Z. Quantum computing for healthcare: a review. Fut Internet. 2023;15(3):94. https://doi.org/10.3390/fi15030094.
10. Durant TJS, Knight E, Nelson B, Dudgeon T, et al. A primer for quantum computing and its applications to healthcare and biomedical research. J Am Med Informatics Assoc. 2024;31(8):1774–84. https://doi.org/10.1093/jamia/ocad093.
11. Li W, Yin Z, Li X, et al. A hybrid quantum computing pipeline for real world drug discovery. Sci Rep. 2024;14(1):Article 16942. https://doi.org/10.1038/s41598-024-67897-8.
12. National Quantum Computing Centre (NQCC). The convergence of healthcare and pharmaceuticals with quantum computing: a new frontier in medicine. (Insights Paper). NQCC/UKRI. Available via NQCC Publications; 2025.

Metaverse and Digital Medicine

13. Wang G, Badal A, Jia X, Maltz JS, Mueller K, Zeng R. Development of metaverse for intelligent healthcare. Nat Mach Intell. 2022;4(12):922–9. https://doi.org/10.1038/s42256-022-00549-6.
14. Hulsen T. Applications of the metaverse in medicine and healthcare. Adv Lab Med. 2024;5(2):159–65. https://doi.org/10.1515/almed-2023-0124.
15. Wang Y, Zhu M, Chen X, Liu R, Ge J, Song Y, Yu G. The application of metaverse in healthcare. Front Public Health. 2024;12:Article 1420367. https://doi.org/10.3389/fpubh.2024.1420367.
16. Kim JH, Lee JH, Kim J, et al. Analyzing usage of the metaverse by associations of patients with prostate cancer during the 2023 Blue Ribbon Campaign: cross-sectional survey. J Med Internet Res. 2025;27(1):e63030. https://doi.org/10.2196/63030.

Appendix F

Cardiology

17. Takahashi EA, et al. An overview of telehealth in the management of cardiovascular disease: a scientific statement from the American Heart Association. Circulation. 2022;146(25):e558–68. https://doi.org/10.1161/CIR.0000000000001107.
18. Kuan PX, et al. Efficacy of telemedicine for the management of cardiovascular disease: a systematic review and meta-analysis. Lancet Digital Health. 2022;4(9):e676–91. https://doi.org/10.1016/S2589-7500(22)00124-8.
19. Huerne K, Eisenberg MJ. Advancing telemedicine in cardiology: a comprehensive review of evolving practices and outcomes in a postpandemic context. Cardiovasc Digit Health J. 2024;5(2):96–110. https://doi.org/10.1016/j.cvdhj.2024.02.001.
20. Tromp J, et al. World heart federation roadmap for digital health in cardiology. Global Heart. 2022;17(1):61. https://doi.org/10.5334/gh.1141.

Endocrinology/Diabetology

21. Moschonis G, et al. Effectiveness, reach, uptake, and feasibility of digital health interventions for adults with Type 2 diabetes: a systematic review and meta-analysis of RCTs. Lancet Digital Health. 2023;5(3):e125–43. https://doi.org/10.1016/S2589-7500(22)00233-3.

22. Udsen FW, et al. The effectiveness of telemedicine solutions in Type 1 diabetes management: a systematic review and meta-analysis. J Diabetes Sci Technol. 2023;17(3):782–93. https://doi.org/10.1177/19322968221076874.
23. Duong T, et al. Digital health interventions to prevent Type 2 diabetes mellitus: systematic review. J Med Internet Res. 2025;27(2025):e67507. https://doi.org/10.2196/67507.
24. Fleming GA, et al. Diabetes digital app technology: benefits, challenges, and recommendations – a consensus report by the ADA and EASD. Diabetes Care. 2020;43(1):250–60. https://doi.org/10.2337/dci19-0062.

Oncology

25. Pennell NA, et al. Telehealth in oncology: ASCO standards and practice recommendations. JCO Oncol Pract. 2021;17(9):546–64. https://doi.org/10.1200/OP.21.00438.
26. Basch E, et al. Overall survival results of a trial assessing patient-reported outcomes for symptom monitoring during routine cancer treatment. JAMA. 2017;318(2):197–8. https://doi.org/10.1001/jama.2017.7156.
27. Borkar S, et al. Revolutionizing oncology: a comprehensive review of digital health applications. Cureus. 2024;16(4):e59203. https://doi.org/10.7759/cureus.59203.
28. Lee K, et al. Digital health interventions for adult patients with cancer evaluated in randomized controlled trials: scoping review. J Med Internet Res. 2023;25(2023):e38333. https://doi.org/10.2196/38333.

Psychiatry/Mental Health

29. Torous J, et al. The evolving field of digital mental health: current evidence and implementation issues for smartphone apps, generative AI, and virtual reality. World Psychiatry. 2025;24(2):156–74. https://doi.org/10.1002/wps.21299.
30. Mucic D, et al. The world psychiatric association telepsychiatry global guidelines. J Technol Behav Sci. 2024;9:572–9. https://doi.org/10.1007/s41347-023-00339-w.
31. Karyotaki E, et al. Internet-based cognitive behavioral therapy for depression: a systematic review and individual patient data network meta-analysis. JAMA Psychiatry. 2021;78(4):361–71. https://doi.org/10.1001/jamapsychiatry.2020.4364.
32. Hollis C, et al. Annual research review: digital health interventions for children and young people with mental health problems – a systematic and meta-review. J Child Psychol Psychiatry. 2017;58(4):474–503. https://doi.org/10.1111/jcpp.12663.

Primary Care

33. Mahdavi S, et al. The use of telemedicine in family medicine: a scoping review. BMC Health Serv Res. 2025;25:376. https://doi.org/10.1186/s12913-025-12449-7.
34. Flodgren G, et al. Interactive telemedicine for managing chronic illness: cochrane review. Cochrane Database Syst Rev. 2015;9:CD007714. https://doi.org/10.1002/14651858.CD007714.pub3.
35. World Health Organization. WHO guideline: recommendations on digital interventions for health system strengthening. Geneva: WHO; 2019. Available from: who.int/publications-detail-redirect/9789241550505
36. Shigekawa E, et al. The current state of telehealth evidence: a rapid review. Health Affairs. 2018;37(12):1975–82. https://doi.org/10.1377/hlthaff.2018.05132.

Pediatrics

37. Curfman AL, et al. Telehealth: improving access to and quality of pediatric health care. Pediatrics. 2022;150(3):e2021056035. https://doi.org/10.1542/peds.2021-056035.
38. Kollins SH, et al. A novel digital intervention for actively reducing severity of paediatric ADHD (STARS-ADHD): a randomised controlled trial. Lancet Digital Health. 2020;2(4):e168–78. https://doi.org/10.1016/S2589-7500(20)30017-0.
39. Curfman AL, et al. Pediatric telehealth in the COVID-19 pandemic era and beyond. Pediatrics. 2021;148(3):e2020047795. https://doi.org/10.1542/peds.2020-047795.
40. Hollis C, et al. Digital health interventions for children and young people with mental health problems – a meta-review. J Child Psychol Psychiatry. 2017;58(4):474–503. https://doi.org/10.1111/jcpp.12663.

Neurology

41. Schwamm LH, et al. Recommendations for the implementation of telehealth in cardiovascular and stroke care: a policy statement from the AHA. Circulation. 2017;135(7):e24–44. https://doi.org/10.1161/CIR.0000000000000475.
42. Hatcher-Martin JM, et al. American academy of neurology telehealth position statement. Neurology. 2021;97(7):334–9. https://doi.org/10.1212/WNL.0000000000012185.
43. Demaerschalk BM, et al. American telemedicine association: telestroke guidelines. Telemed J E Health. 2017;23(5):376–89. https://doi.org/10.1089/tmj.2017.0006.
44. León-Salas B, et al. Telemedicine for neurological diseases: a systematic review and meta-analysis. Eur J Neurol. 2023;30(1):241–54. https://doi.org/10.1111/ene.15599.

Rheumatology

45. de Thurah A, et al. 2022 EULAR points to consider for remote care in rheumatic and musculoskeletal diseases. Ann Rheumat Dis. 2022;81(8):1065–71. https://doi.org/10.1136/annrheumdis-2022-222341.
46. Marques A, et al. Telehealth for patients with rheumatic diseases: systematic review informing the 2022 EULAR recommendations. RMD Open. 2022;8(2):e002387. https://doi.org/10.1136/rmdopen-2022-002387.
47. Venuturupalli S, et al. Home-based telemedicine in rheumatology – a scoping review. ACR Open Rheumatol. 2024;6(5):312–20. https://doi.org/10.1002/acr2.11660.
48. Wood PR, et al. Telemedicine in rheumatology: during and beyond COVID-19. Curr Opin Rheumatol. 2021;33(3):263–9. https://doi.org/10.1097/BOR.0000000000000796.

Infectious Diseases

49. Craig KJT, et al. Effectiveness of contact tracing for viral disease mitigation and suppression: evidence-based review. JMIR Public Health Surveill. 2021;7(10):e32468. https://doi.org/10.2196/32468.
50. World Health Organization. Ethical considerations in the use of digital proximity tracking technologies for COVID-19 contact tracing. WHO Policy Brief, 2020. Available at: who.int/publications/i/item/WHO-2019-nCoV-Ethics_Contact_tracing-2020.1
51. Subbaraman R, et al. Effect of digital adherence technologies on tuberculosis treatment outcomes in India: a randomized trial. Lancet. 2021;398(10315):1612–24. https://doi.org/10.1016/S0140-6736(21)00436-6.

52. Harden SM, et al. Implementation of digital contact tracing and remote monitoring for infectious diseases: lessons from COVID-19. J Infect Dis. 2022;225(Suppl 1):S108–17. https://doi.org/10.1093/infdis/jiab554.

Pulmonology

53. Koh JH, et al. Telemedical interventions for chronic obstructive pulmonary disease management: umbrella review. J Med Internet Res. 2023;25(2023):e38057. https://doi.org/10.2196/38057.
54. McLean S, et al. Telehealthcare for chronic obstructive pulmonary disease: cochrane review and meta-analysis. Br J Gen Pract. 2012;62(604):e739–47. https://doi.org/10.3399/bjgp12X658269.
55. Laver KE, et al. Telerehabilitation services for stroke, COPD, heart failure and coronary disease: an evidence and gap map. Cochrane Database Syst Rev. 2020;11:CD013632. https://doi.org/10.1002/14651858.CD013632.
56. Alrajhi KN, et al. Effectiveness of telemonitoring for reducing COPD exacerbations: a systematic review and meta-analysis. Front Med. 2022;9:888941. https://doi.org/10.3389/fmed.2022.888941.

Rehabilitation

57. Hao J, et al. Effects of virtual reality–based telerehabilitation for stroke patients: a systematic review and meta-analysis of RCTs. J Stroke Cerebrovasc Dis. 2023;32(3):106960. https://doi.org/10.1016/j.jstrokecerebrovasdis.2022.106960.
58. Chen J, et al. Telerehabilitation approaches for stroke: systematic review and meta-analysis of functional outcomes. Arch Phys Med Rehabil. 2020;101(2):359–73. https://doi.org/10.1016/j.apmr.2019.08.482.
59. Cottrell MA, et al. Telehealth for musculoskeletal rehabilitation: systematic review and meta-analysis. J Telemed Telecare. 2017;23(2):212–21. https://doi.org/10.1177/1357633X16643796.
60. Prvu Bettger J, et al. Effect of virtual home rehabilitation on functional outcomes after hospitalization for stroke: a randomized clinical trial. JAMA Neurol. 2020;77(11):1470–8. https://doi.org/10.1001/jamaneurol.2020.2896.

Dermatology

61. Tensen E, et al. Two decades of teledermatology: current status and integration in national healthcare systems. Curr Dermatol Rep. 2020;9(1):1–11. https://doi.org/10.1007/s13671-020-00289-6.
62. Phillips M, et al. Assessment of accuracy of an artificial intelligence algorithm to detect melanoma in images of skin lesions. JAMA Network Open. 2019;2(10):e1913436. https://doi.org/10.1001/jamanetworkopen.2019.13436.
63. Barbieri JS, et al. Telemedicine for skin disease. JAMA. 2020;324(2):152–3. https://doi.org/10.1001/jama.2020.7091.
64. Young PM, et al. Teledermatology: a review of image quality, diagnosis, and management. Dermatol Clin. 2021;39(4):491–8. https://doi.org/10.1016/j.det.2021.05.001.

Geriatrics

65. Masterson Creber RM, et al. Telehealth and health equity in older adults with heart failure: a scientific statement from the AHA. Circ Cardiovasc Qual Outcomes. 2023;16(11):e000123. https://doi.org/10.1161/HCQ.0000000000000123.
66. Kvedar JC, et al. Connected health and the digital aging revolution. Ageing Res Rev. 2020;62:101110. https://doi.org/10.1016/j.arr.2020.101110.
67. Seifert A, et al. The digital divide in older adults: existing evidence and research directions. Gerontologist. 2020;60(1):26–32. https://doi.org/10.1093/geront/gnz102.
68. Levy CR, et al. Virtual care for geriatric fracture management: opportunities and challenges. J Am Acad Orthop Surg. 2022;30(1):e22–9. https://doi.org/10.5435/JAAOS-D-21-00547.

Nephrology

69. Chan L, et al. Outcomes of remote patient management in automated peritoneal dialysis: a cluster randomized trial. J Am Soc Nephrol. 2021;32(5):1235–46. https://doi.org/10.1681/ASN.2020081187.
70. Ishani A, et al. Telehealth by an interprofessional team in patients with CKD: a randomized controlled trial. Am J Kidney Dis. 2016;68(1):41–9. https://doi.org/10.1053/j.ajkd.2015.12.028.
71. Subramanian L, et al. Remote monitoring in home-based peritoneal dialysis: a systematic review. Clin J Am Soc Nephrol. 2019;12(12):2000–13. https://doi.org/10.2215/CJN.08360819.
72. Radhakrishnan J, Budianto I. Digital health in nephrology: promises and pitfalls. Kidney360. 2021;2(5):832–41. https://doi.org/10.34067/KID.0000132021.

Gastroenterology

73. Atreja A, et al. Digital health in gastroenterology: path to transformation. Gastroenterology. 2018;154(6):1772–4. https://doi.org/10.1053/j.gastro.2018.03.067.
74. Dixon BE, et al. An informatics approach to medication adherence assessment and improvement using clinical electronic records. J Am Med Inform Assoc. 2016;23(3):621–8. https://doi.org/10.1093/jamia/ocv164.
75. Deen J, et al. Telemedicine in hepatology: current status and future perspectives. J Clin Transl Hepatol. 2020;8(4):413–23. https://doi.org/10.14218/JCTH.2020.00036.
76. Nielepkowicz J, et al. Artificial intelligence in gastrointestinal endoscopy: a state-of-the-art review. Clin Res Hepatol Gastroenterol. 2023;47(2):102058. https://doi.org/10.1016/j.clinre.2022.102058.

Surgery

77. Wanees F, et al. Bridging distances and enhancing care: a comprehensive review of telemedicine in surgery. Cureus. 2025;17(1):e38000. https://doi.org/10.7759/cureus.38000.
78. Pinto A, et al. Telemedicine and robotic surgery: a narrative review of advantages, limitations, and future developments. Electronics. 2023;13(1):124. https://doi.org/10.3390/electronics13010124.
79. Rojas-Muñoz E, et al. Telesurgery's evolution during the robotic surgery renaissance: an ethical and systematic review. Surg Innov. 2021;28(2):210–9. https://doi.org/10.1177/1553350620977029.
80. Yang XF, Wang P. Augmented reality–assisted surgery: applications, promises, and challenges. Int J Surg. 2020;79:169–79. https://doi.org/10.1016/j.ijsu.2020.05.050.

Index

A. Cesario et al., *Digital Medicine Starter Guide*,
https://doi.org/10.1007/978-3-032-01272-2

K

L

M

N

O

P

MIX
Papier aus verantwortungsvollen Quellen
Paper from responsible sources
FSC® C105338

If you have any concerns about our products, you can contact us on
ProductSafety@springernature.com

In case Publisher is established outside the EU, the EU authorized representative is:
Springer Nature Customer Service Center GmbH
Europaplatz 3, 69115 Heidelberg, Germany

Printed by Libri Plureos GmbH
in Hamburg, Germany